Vets Might Fly

James Herriot grew up in Glasgow and qualified as a veterinary surgeon at Glasgow Veterinary College. Shortly afterwards he took up a position as an assistant in a North Yorkshire practice where he has remained, with the exception of his wartime service in the RAF (in part the subject of this book).

James Herriot's interests extend beyond writing and veterinary work to music, and dog-walking in the Dales. He is married, with a son who is also a veterinary surgeon and a daughter who is a doctor.

James Herriot is a pseudonym.

Previously published by
James Herriot in Pan Books

If Only They Could Talk
It Shouldn't Happen to a Vet
Let Sleeping Vets Lie
Vet in Harness

All Creatures Great and Small
(an omnibus edition comprising the
first two titles above and part of the third)

James Herriot

Vets Might Fly

Pan Books London and Sydney

The four lines from *If I Only Had Wings* on p. 78 are reproduced by permission of The Peter Maurice Music Co Ltd, 138–140 Charing Cross Road, London WC2H OLD, England

First published in Great Britain 1976 by Michael Joseph Ltd
This edition published 1977 by Pan Books Ltd,
Cavaye Place, London SW10 9PG
© James Herriot 1976
ISBN 0 330 25221 6
Printed and bound in Great Britain by
Richard Clay (The Chaucer Press) Ltd, Bungay, Suffolk

to my dogs,
Hector and **Dan**
faithful companions of the daily round

one

'Move!' bawled the drill corporal. 'Come on, speed it up!'
He sprinted effortlessly to the rear of the gasping, panting
column of men and urged us on from there.

I was somewhere in the middle, jog-trotting laboriously
with the rest and wondering how much longer I could keep
going. And as my ribs heaved agonizingly and my leg
muscles protested, I tried to work out just how many miles
we had run.

I had suspected nothing when we lined up outside our
billets. We weren't clad in PT kit but in woollen pullovers and
regulation slacks and it seemed unlikely that anything violent
was imminent. The corporal, too, a cheerful little cockney,
appeared to regard us as his brothers. He had a kind face.

'Awright, lads,' he had cried, smiling over the fifty new
airmen. 'We're just going to trot round to the park, so
follow me. Le-eft turn! At the double, qui-ick march!
'eft-ight, 'eft-ight, 'eft-ight!'

That had been a long, long time ago and we were still
reeling through the London streets with never a sign of a
park anywhere. The thought hammered in my brain that I
had been under the impression that I was fit. A country vet,
especially in the Yorkshire Dales, never had the chance to
get out of condition; he was always on the move, wrestling
with the big animals, walking for miles between the fell-side
barns; he was hard and tough. That's what I thought.

But now other reflections began to creep in. My few
months of married life with Helen had been so much lotus
eating. She was too good a cook and I was too faithful a
disciple of her art. Just lounging by our bed-sitter's fireside
was the sweetest of all occupations. I had tried to ignore the
disappearance of my abdominal muscles, the sagging of my
pectorals, but it was all coming home to me now.

'It's not far now, lads,' the corporal chirped from the rear,
but he struck no responsive chords in the toiling group. He

had said it several times before and we had stopped believing him.

But this time it seemed he really meant it, because as we turned into yet another street I could see iron railings and trees at the far end. The relief was inexpressible. I would just about have the strength to make it through the gates – to the rest and smoke which I badly needed because my legs were beginning to seize up.

We passed under an arch of branches which still bore a few autumn leaves and stopped as one man, but the corporal was waving us on.

'Come on, lads, round the track!' he shouted and pointed to a broad earthen path which circled the park.

We stared at him. He couldn't be serious! A storm of protest broke out.

'Aw no, corp . . . !' 'Have a heart, corp . . . !'

The smile vanished from the little man's face. 'Get movin', I said! Faster, faster . . . one-two, one-two.'

As I stumbled forward over the black earth, between borders of sooty rhododendrons and tired grass, I just couldn't believe it. It was all too sudden. Three days ago I was in Darrowby and half of me was still back there, back with Helen. And another part was still looking out of the rear window of the taxi at the green hills receding behind the tiled roofs into the morning sunshine; still standing in the corridor of the train as the flat terrain of southern England slid past and a great weight built up steadily in my chest.

My first introduction to the RAF was at Lord's cricket ground. Masses of forms to fill, medicals, then the issue of an enormous pile of kit. I was billeted in a block of flats in St John's Wood – luxurious before the lush fittings had been removed. But they couldn't take away the heavy bathroom ware and one of our blessings was the unlimited hot water gushing at our touch into the expensive surroundings.

After that first crowded day I retired to one of those green-tiled sanctuaries and lathered myself with a new bar of a famous toilet soap which Helen had put in my bag. I have never been able to use that soap since. Scents are too evocative and the merest whiff jerks me back to that first night away from my wife, and to the feeling I had then. It was a dull, empty ache which never really went away.

On the second day we marched endlessly; lectures, meals, inoculations. I was used to syringes but the very sight of them was too much for many of my friends. Especially when the doctor took the blood samples; one look at the dark fluid flowing from their veins and the young men toppled quietly from their chairs, often four or five in a row while the orderlies, grinning cheerfully, bore them away.

We ate in the London Zoo and our meals were made interesting by the chatter of monkeys and the roar of lions in the background. But in between it was march, march, march, with our new boots giving us hell.

And on this third day the whole thing was still a blur. We had been wakened as on my first morning by the hideous 6 a.m. clattering of dustbin lids; I hadn't really expected a bugle but I found this noise intolerable. However, at the moment my only concern was that we had completed the circuit of the park. The gates were only a few yards ahead and I staggered up to them and halted among my groaning comrades.

'Round again, lads!' the corporal yelled, and as we stared at him aghast he smiled affectionately. 'You think this is tough? Wait till they get hold of you at ITW. I'm just kinda breakin' you in gently. You'll thank me for this later. Right, at the double! One-two, one-two!'

Bitter thoughts assailed me as I lurched forward once more. Another round of the park would kill me – there was not a shadow of a doubt about that. You left a loving wife and a happy home to serve king and country and this was how they treated you. It wasn't fair

The night before I had dreamed of Darrowby. I was back in old Mr Dakin's cow byre. The farmer's patient eyes in the long, drooping-moustached face looked down at me from his stooping height.

'It looks as though it's over wi' awd Blossom, then,' he

said, and rested his hand briefly on the old cow's back. It was an enormous, work-swollen hand. Mr Dakin's gaunt frame carried little flesh but the grossly thickened fingers bore testimony to a life of toil.

I dried off the needle and dropped it into the metal box where I carried my suture materials, scalpels and blades. 'Well, it's up to you of course, Mr Dakin, but this is the third time I've had to stitch her teats and I'm afraid it's going to keep on happening.'

'Aye, it's just the shape she is.' The farmer bent and examined the row of knots along the four-inch scar. 'By gaw, you wouldn't believe it could mek such a mess – just another cow standin' on it.'

'A cow's hoof is sharp,' I said. 'It's nearly like a knife coming down.'

That was the worst of very old cows. Their udders dropped and their teats became larger and more pendulous so that when they lay down in their stalls the vital milk-producing organ was pushed away to one side into the path of the neighbouring animals. If it wasn't Mabel on the right standing on it, it was Buttercup on the other side.

There were only six cows in the little cobbled byre with its low roof and wooden partitions and they all had names. You don't find cows with names any more and there aren't any farmers like Mr Dakin, who somehow scratched a living from a herd of six milkers plus a few calves, pigs and hens.

'Aye, well,' he said. 'Ah reckon t'awd lass doesn't owe me anythin'. Ah remember the night she was born, twelve years ago. She was out of awd Daisy and ah carried her out of this very byre on a sack and the snow was comin' down hard. Sin' then ah wouldn't like to count how many thousand gallons o' milk she's turned out – she's still givin' four a day. Naw, she doesn't owe me a thing.'

As if she knew she was the topic of conversation Blossom turned her head and looked at him. She was the classical picture of an ancient bovine; as fleshless as her owner, with jutting pelvic bones, splayed, overgrown feet and horns with a multitude of rings along their curving length. Beneath her, the udder, once high and tight, drooped forlornly almost to the floor.

She resembled her owner, too, in her quiet, patient demeanour. I had infiltrated her teat with a local anaesthetic before stitching but I don't think she would have moved if I hadn't used any. Stitching teats puts a vet in the ideal position to be kicked, with his head low down in front of the hind feet, but there was no danger with Blossom. She had never kicked anybody in her life.

Mr Dakin blew out his cheeks. 'Well, there's nowt else for it. She'll have to go. I'll tell Jack Dodson to pick 'er up for the fatstock market on Thursday. She'll be a bit tough for eatin' but ah reckon she'll make a few steak pies.'

He was trying to joke but he was unable to smile as he looked at the old cow. Behind him, beyond the open door, the green hillside ran down to the river and the spring sunshine touched the broad sweep of the shallows with a million dancing lights. A beach of bleached stones gleamed bone-white against the long stretch of grassy bank which rolled up to the pastures lining the valley floor.

I had often felt that this smallholding would be an ideal place to live; only a mile outside Darrowby, but secluded, and with this heart-lifting vista of river and fell. I remarked on this once to Mr Dakin and the old man turned to me with a wry smile.

'Aye, but the view's not very sustainin',' he said.

It happened that I was called back to the farm on the following Thursday to 'cleanse' a cow and was in the byre when Dodson the drover called to pick up Blossom. He had collected a group of fat bullocks and cows from other farms and they stood, watched by one of his men, on the road high above.

'Nah then, Mr Dakin,' he cried as he bustled in. 'It's easy to see which one you want me to tek. It's that awd screw over there.'

He pointed at Blossom, and in truth the unkind description seemed to fit the bony creature standing between her sleek neighbours.

The farmer did not reply for a moment, then he went up between the cows and gently rubbed Blossom's forehead. 'Aye, this is the one, Jack.' He hesitated, then undid the chain round her neck. 'Off ye go, awd lass,' he murmured, and the old animal turned and made her way placidly from the stall.

'Aye, come on with ye!' shouted the dealer, poking his stick against the cow's rump.

'Doan't hit 'er!' barked Mr Dakin.

Dodson looked at him in surprise. 'Ah never 'it 'em, you know that. Just send 'em on, like,'

'Ah knaw, ah knaw, Jack, but you won't need your stick for this 'un. She'll go wherever ye want – allus has done.'

Blossom confirmed his words as she ambled through the door and, at a gesture from the farmer, turned along the track.

The old man and I stood watching as the cow made her way unhurriedly up the hill, Jack Dodson in his long khaki smock sauntering behind her. As the path wound behind a clump of sparse trees man and beast disappeared but Mr Dakin still gazed after them, listening to the clip-clop of the hooves on the hard ground.

When the sound died away he turned to me quickly. 'Right, Mr Herriot, we'll get on wi' our job, then. I'll bring your hot watter.'

The farmer was silent as I soaped my arm and inserted it into the cow. If there is one thing more disagreeable than removing the bovine afterbirth it is watching somebody else doing it, and I always try to maintain a conversation as I grope around inside. But this time it was hard work. Mr Dakin responded to my sallies on the weather, cricket and the price of milk with a series of grunts.

Holding the cow's tail he leaned on the hairy back and, empty-eyed, blew smoke from the pipe which like most farmers at a cleansing he had prudently lit at the outset. And of course, since the going was heavy, it just would happen that the job took much longer than usual. Sometimes a placenta simply lifted out but I had this one away from the cotyledons one by one, returning every few minutes to the hot water and antiseptic to re-soap my aching arms.

But at last it was finished. I pushed in a couple of pessaries, untied the sack from my middle and pulled my shirt over my head. The conversation had died and the silence was almost oppressive as we opened the byre door.

Mr Dakin paused, his hand on the latch. 'What's that?' he said softly.

From somewhere on the hillside I could hear the clip-clop of a cow's feet. There were two ways to the farm and the sound came from a narrow track which joined the main road half a mile beyond the other entrance. As we listened a cow rounded a rocky outcrop and came towards us.

It was Blossom, moving at a brisk trot, great udder swinging, eyes fixed purposefully on the open door behind us.

'What the hangment . . . ?' Mr Dakin burst out, but the old cow brushed past us and marched without hesitation into the stall which she had occupied for all those years. She sniffed enquiringly at the empty hay rack and looked round at her owner.

Mr Dakin stared back at her. The eyes in the weathered face were expressionless but the smoke rose from his pipe in a series of rapid puffs.

Heavy boots clattered suddenly outside and Jack Dodson panted his way through the door.

'Oh, you're there, ye awd beggar!' he gasped. 'Ah thought I'd lost ye!'

He turned to the farmer. 'By gaw, I'm sorry, Mr Dakin. She must 'ave turned off at t'top of your other path. Ah never saw her go.'

The farmer shrugged. 'It's awright, Jack. It's not your fault, ah should've told ye.'

'That's soon mended anyway.' The drover grinned and moved towards Blossom. 'Come on, lass, let's have ye out o' there again.'

But he halted as Mr Dakin held an arm in front of him.

There was a long silence as Dodson and I looked in surprise at the farmer who continued to gaze fixedly at the cow. There was a pathetic dignity about the old animal as she stood there against the mouldering timber of the partition, her eyes patient and undemanding. It was a dignity which triumphed over the unsightliness of the long upturned hooves, the fleshless ribs, the broken-down udder almost brushing the cobbles.

Then, still without speaking, Mr Dakin moved unhurriedly between the cows and a faint chink of metal sounded as he fastened the chain around Blossom's neck. Then he strolled to the end of the byre and returned with a forkful of hay which he tossed expertly into the rack.

This was what Blossom was waiting for. She jerked a mouthful from between the spars and began to chew with quiet satisfaction.

'What's to do, Mr Dakin?' the drover cried in bewilderment. 'They're waiting for me at t'mart!'

The farmer tapped out his pipe on the half door and began to fill it with black shag from a battered tin. 'Ah'm sorry to waste your time, Jack, but you'll have to go without 'er.'

'Without 'er . . . ? But . . . ?'

'Aye, ye'll think I'm daft, but that's how it is. T'awd lass has come 'ome and she's stoppin' 'ome.' He directed a look of flat finality at the drover.

Dodson nodded a couple of times then shuffled from the byre. Mr Dakin followed and called after him.

'Ah'll pay ye for your time, Jack. Put it down on ma bill.'

He returned, applied a match to his pipe and drew deeply.

'Mr Herriot,' he said as the smoke rose around his ears, 'do you ever feel when summat happens that it was meant to happen and that it was for t'best?'

'Yes, I do, Mr Dakin. I often feel that.'

'Aye well, that's how I felt when Blossom came down that hill.' He reached out and scratched the root of the cow's tail. 'She's allus been a favourite and by gaw I'm glad she's back.'

'But how about those teats? I'm willing to keep stitching them up, but. . . .'

'Nay, lad, ah've had an idea. Just came to me when you

were tekkin' away that cleansin' and I thowt I was ower late.'

'An idea?'

'Aye.' The old man nodded and tamped down the tobacco with his thumb. 'I can put two or three calves on to 'er instead of milkin' 'er. The old stable is empty – she can live in there where there's nobody to stand on 'er awd tits.'

I laughed. 'You're right, Mr Dakin. She'd be safe in the stable and she'd suckle three calves easily. She could pay her way.'

'Well, as ah said, it's matterless. After all them years she doesn't owe me a thing.' A gentle smile spread over the seamed face. 'Main thing is, she's come 'ome.'

My eyes were shut most of the time now as I blundered round the park and when I opened them a red mist swirled. But it is incredible what the human frame will stand and I blinked in disbelief as the iron gates appeared once more under their arch of sooty branches.

I had survived the second lap but an ordinary rest would be inadequate now. This time I would have to lie down. I felt sick.

'Good lads!' the corporal called out, cheerful as ever. 'You're doin' fine. Now we're just going to 'ave a little hoppin' on the spot.'

Incredulous wails rose from our demoralized band but the corporal was unabashed.

'Feet together now. Up! Up! Up! That's no good, come on, get some height into it! Up! Up!'

This was the final absurdity. My chest was a flaming cavern of agony. These people were supposed to be making us fit and instead they were doing irreparable damage to my heart and lungs.

'You'll thank me for this later, lads. Take my word for it. GET YOURSELVES OFF THE GROUND. UP! UP!'

Through my pain I could see the corporal's laughing face. The man was clearly a sadist. It was no good appealing to him.

And as, with the last of my strength, I launched myself into the air it came to me suddenly why I had dreamed about Blossom last night.

I wanted to go home, too.

two

The fog swirled over the heads of the marching men; a London fog, thick, yellow, metallic on the tongue. I couldn't see the head of the column, only the swinging lantern carried by the leader.

This 6.30 a.m. walk to breakfast was just about the worst part of the day, when my morale was low and thoughts of home rose painfully.

We used to have fogs in Darrowby, but they were country fogs, different from this. One morning I drove out on my rounds with the headlights blazing against the grey curtain ahead, seeing nothing from my tight-shut box. But I was heading up the Dale, climbing steadily with the engine pulling against the rising ground, then quite suddenly the fog thinned to a shimmering silvery mist and was gone.

And there, above the pall, the sun was dazzling and the long green line of the fells rose before me, thrusting exultantly into a sky of summer blue.

Spellbound, I drove upwards into the bright splendour, staring through the windscreen as though I had never seen it all before; the bronze of the dead bracken spilling down the grassy flanks of the hills, the dark smudges of trees, the grey farmhouses and the endless pattern of walls creeping to the heather above.

I was in a rush as usual but I had to stop. I pulled up in a gateway, Sam jumped out and we went through into a field; and as the beagle scampered over the glittering turf I stood in the warm sunshine amid the melting frost and looked back at the dark damp blanket which blotted out the low country but left this jewelled world above it.

And, gulping the sweet air, I gazed about me gratefully at the clean green land where I worked and made my living.

I could have stayed there, wandering round, watching Sam exploring with waving tail, nosing into the shady corners where the sun had not reached and the ground was iron hard and the rime thick and crisp on the grass. But I had an appointment to keep, and no ordinary one – it was with a peer of the realm. Reluctantly I got back into the car.

I was due to start Lord Hulton's tuberculin test at 9.30 a.m. and as I drove round the back of the Elizabethan mansion to the farm buildings nearby I felt a pang of misgiving; there were no animals in sight. There was only a man in tattered blue dungarees hammering busily at a makeshift crush at the exit to the fold yard.

He turned round when he saw me and waved his hammer. As I approached I looked wonderingly at the slight figure with the soft fairish hair falling over his brow, at the holed cardigan and muck-encrusted wellingtons. You would have expected him to say, 'Nah then, Mr Herriot, how ista this mornin'?'

But he didn't, he said, 'Herriot, my dear chap, I'm most frightfully sorry, but I'm very much afraid we're not quite ready for you.' And he began to fumble with his tobacco pouch.

William George Henry Augustus, Eleventh Marquis of Hulton, always had a pipe in his mouth and he was invariably either filling it, cleaning it out with a metal reaming tool or trying to light it. I had never seen him actually smoking it. And at times of stress he attempted to do everything at once. He was obviously embarrassed at his lack of preparedness and when he saw me glance involuntarily at my watch he grew more agitated, pulling his pipe from his mouth and putting it back in again, tucking the hammer under his arm, rummaging in a large box of matches.

I gazed across to the rising ground beyond the farm buildings. Far off on the horizon I could make out tiny figures: galloping beasts, scurrying men; and faint sounds came down to me of barking dogs, irritated bellowings and shrill cries of 'Haow, haow!' 'Gerraway by!' 'Siddown, dog!'

I sighed. It was the old story. Even the Yorkshire aristocracy seemed to share this carefree attitude to time.

His lordship clearly sensed my feelings because his discomfort increased.

'It's too bad of me, old chap,' he said, spraying a few matchsticks around and dropping flakes of tobacco on the stone flags. 'I did promise to be ready for nine thirty but those blasted animals just won't cooperate.'

I managed a smile. 'Oh never mind, Lord Hulton, they seem to be getting them down the hill now and I'm not in such a panic this morning, anyway.'

'Oh splendid, splendid!' He attempted to ignite a towering mound of dark flake which spluttered feebly then toppled over the edge of his pipe. 'And come and see this! I've been rigging up a crush. We'll drive them in here and we'll really have 'em. Remember we had a spot of bother last time, what?'

I nodded. I did remember. Lord Hulton had only about thirty suckling cows but it had taken a three-hour rodeo to test them. I looked doubtfully at the rickety structure of planks and corrugated iron. It would be interesting to see how it coped with the moorland cattle.

I didn't mean to rub it in, but again I glanced unthinkingly at my watch and the little man winced as though he had received a blow.

'Dammit!' he burst out. 'What are they doing over there? Tell you what, I'll go and give them a hand!' Distractedly, he began to change hammer, pouch, pipe and matches from hand to hand, dropping them and picking them up, before finally deciding to put the hammer down and stuff the rest into his pockets. He went off at a steady trot and I thought as I had done so often that there couldn't be many noblemen in England like him.

If I had been a marquis, I felt, I would still have been in

bed or perhaps just parting the curtains and peering out to see what kind of day it was. But Lord Hulton worked all the time, just about as hard as any of his men. One morning I arrived to find him at the supremely mundane task of 'plugging muck', standing on a manure heap, hurling steaming forkfuls on to a cart. And he always dressed in rags. I suppose he must have had more orthodox items in his wardrobe but I never saw them. Even his tobacco was the great smoke of the ordinary farmer – Redbreast Flake.

My musings were interrupted by the thunder of hooves and wild cries; the Hulton herd was approaching. Within minutes the fold yard was filled with milling creatures, steam rising in rolling clouds from their bodies.

The marquis appeared round the corner of the building at a gallop.

'Right, Charlie!' he yelled. 'Let the first one into the crush!'

Panting with anticipation he stood by the nailed boards as the men inside opened the yard gate. He didn't have to wait long. A shaggy red monster catapulted from the interior, appeared briefly in the narrow passage then emerged at about fifty miles an hour from the other end with portions of his lordship's creation dangling from its horns and neck. The rest of the herd pounded close behind.

'Stop them! Stop them!' screamed the little peer, but it was of no avail. A hairy torrent flooded through the opening and in no time at all the herd was legging it back to the high land in a wild stampede. The men followed them and within a few moments Lord Hulton and I were standing there just as before watching the tiny figures on the skyline, listening to the distant 'Haow, haow!' 'Gerraway by!'

'I say,' he murmured despondently. 'It didn't work terribly well, did it?'

But he was made of stern stuff. Seizing his hammer he began to bang away with undiminished enthusiasm and by the time the beasts returned the crush was rebuilt and a stout iron bar pushed across the front to prevent further break-outs.

It seemed to solve the problem because the first cow, confronted by the bar, stood quietly and I was able to clip the hair on her neck through an opening between the planks. Lord Hulton, in high good humour, settled down on an upturned oil drum with my testing book on his knee.

'I'll do the writing for you,' he cried. 'Fire away, old chap!'

I poised my calipers. 'Eight, eight.' He wrote it down and the next cow came in.

'Eight, eight,' I said, and he bowed his head again.

The third cow arrived: 'Eight, eight.' And the fourth, 'Eight, eight.'

His lordship looked up from the book and passed a weary hand across his forehead.

'Herriot, dear boy, can't you vary it a bit? I'm beginning to lose interest.'

All went well until we saw the cow which had originally smashed the crush. She had sustained a slight scratch on her neck.

'I say, look at that!' cried the peer. 'Will it be all right?'

'Oh yes, it's nothing. Superficial.'

'Ah, good, but don't you think we should have something to put on it? Some of that. . . .'

I waited for it. Lord Hulton was a devotee of May and Baker's Propamidine Cream and used it for all minor cuts and grazes in his cattle. He loved the stuff. But unfortunately he couldn't say 'Propamidine'. In fact nobody on the entire establishment could say it except Charlie the farm foreman and he only thought he could say it. He called it 'Propopamide' but his lordship had the utmost faith in him.

'Charlie!' he bawled. 'Are you there, Charlie?'

The foreman appeared from the pack in the yard and touched his cap. 'Yes, m'lord.'

'Charlie, that wonderful stuff we get from Mr Herriot – you know, for cut teats and things. Pro . . . Pero . . . what the hell do you call it again?'

Charlie paused. It was one of his big moments. 'Propopamide, m'lord.'

The marquis, intensely gratified, slapped the knee of his

dungarees. 'That's it, Propopamide! Damned if I can get my tongue round it. Well done, Charlie!'

Charlie inclined his head modestly.

The whole test was a vast improvement on last time and we were finished within an hour and a half. There was just one tragedy. About half way through, one of the cows dropped down dead with an attack of hypomagnesaemia, a condition which often plagues sucklers. It was a sudden, painless collapse and I had no chance to do anything.

Lord Hulton looked down at the animal which had just stopped breathing. 'Do you think we could salvage her for meat if we bled her?'

'Well, it's typical hypomag. Nothing to harm anybody . . . you could try. It would depend on what the meat inspector says.'

The cow was bled, pulled into a van and the peer drove off to the abattoir. He came back just as we were finishing the test.

'How did you get on?' I asked him. 'Did they accept her?'

He hesitated. 'No . . . no, old chap,' he said sadly. 'I'm afraid they didn't.'

'Why? Did the meat inspector condemn the carcass?'

'Well . . . I never got as far as the meat inspector, actually . . . just saw one of the slaughtermen.'

'And what did he say?'

'Just two words, Herriot.'

'Two words . . . ?'

'Yes . . . "Bugger off!" '

I nodded. 'I see.' It was easy to imagine the scene. The tough slaughterman viewing the small, unimpressive figure and deciding that he wasn't going to be put out of his routine by some ragged farm man.

'Well, never mind, sir,' I said. 'You can only try.'

'True . . . true, old chap.' He dropped a few matches as he fumbled disconsolately with his smoking equipment.

As I was getting into the car I remembered about the Propamidine. 'Don't forget to call down for that cream, will you?'

'By Jove, yes! I'll come down for it after lunch. I have great faith in that Prom ... Pram ... Charlie! Damn and blast, what is it?'

Charlie drew himself up proudly. 'Propopamide, m'lord.'

'Ah yes, Propopamide!' The little man laughed, his good humour quite restored. 'Good lad, Charlie, you're a marvel!'

'Thank you, m'lord.' The foreman wore the smug expression of the expert as he drove the cattle back into the field.

It's a funny thing, but when you see a client about something you very often see him soon again about something else. It was only a week later, with the district still in the iron grip of winter, that my bedside phone jangled me from slumber.

After that first palpitation of the heart which I feel does vets no good at all I reached a sleepy hand from under the sheets.

'Yes?' I grunted.

'Herriot ... I say, Herriot ... is that you, Herriot?' The voice was laden with tension.

'Yes, it is, Lord Hulton.'

'Oh good ... good ... dash it, I do apologize. Frightfully bad show, waking you up like this ... but I've got something damn peculiar here.' A soft pattering followed which I took to be matches falling around the receiver.

'Really?' I yawned and my eyes closed involuntarily. 'In what way, exactly?'

'Well, I've been sitting up with one of my best sows. Been farrowing and produced twelve nice piglets, but there's something very odd.'

'How do you mean?'

'Difficult to describe, old chap ... but you know the ... er ... bottom aperture ... there's a bloody great long red thing hanging from it.'

My eyes snapped open and my mouth gaped in a soundless scream. Prolapsed uterus! Hard labour in cows, a pleasant exercise in ewes, impossible in sows.

'Long red ... ! When ... ? How ... ?' I was stammering pointlessly. I didn't have to ask.

'Just popped it out, dear boy. I was waiting for another piglet and whoops, there it was. Gave me a nasty turn.'

My toes curled tightly beneath the blankets. It was no good telling him that I had seen five prolapsed uteri in pigs in my limited experience and had failed in every case. I had come to the conclusion that there was no way of putting them back.

But I had to try. 'I'll be right out,' I muttered.

I looked at the alarm clock. It was five thirty. A horrible time, truncating the night's slumber yet eliminating any chance of a soothing return to bed for an hour before the day's work. And I hated turning out even more since my marriage. Helen was lovely to come back to, but by the same token it was a bigger wrench to leave her soft warm presence and venture into the inhospitable world outside.

And the journey to the Hulton farm was not enlivened by my memories of those five other sows. I had tried everything; full anaesthesia, lifting them upside down with pulleys, directing a jet from a hose on the everted organ, and all the time pushing, straining sweating over the great mass of flesh which refused to go back through that absurdly small hole. The result in each case had been the conversion of my patient into pork pies and a drastic plummeting of my self-esteem.

There was no moon and the soft glow from the piggery door made the only light among the black outlines of the buildings. Lord Hulton was waiting at the entrance and I thought I had better warn him.

'I have to tell you, sir, that this is a very serious condition. It's only fair that you should know that the sow very often has to be slaughtered.'

The little man's eyes widened and the corners of his mouth drooped.

'Oh, I say! That's rather a bore . . . one of my best animals. I . . . I'm rather attached to that pig.' He was wearing a polonecked sweater of such advanced dilapidation that the hem hung in long woollen fronds almost to his knees, and as he tremblingly attempted to light his pipe he looked very vulnerable.

'But I'll do my very best,' I added hastily. 'There's always a chance.'

'Oh, good man!' In his relief, he dropped his pouch and as he stooped the open box of matches spilled around his feet. It was some time before we retrieved them and went into the piggery.

The reality was as bad as my imaginings. Under the single weak electric bulb of the pen an unbelievable length of very solid-looking red tissue stretched from the rear end of a massive white sow lying immobile on her side. The twelve pink piglets fought and worried along the row of teats; they didn't seem to be getting much.

As I stripped off and dipped my arms into the steaming bucket I wished with all my heart that the porcine uterus was a little short thing and not this horrible awkward shape. And it was a disquieting thought that tonight I had no artificial aids. People used all sorts of tricks and various types of equipment but here in this silent building there was just the pig, Lord Hulton and me. His lordship, I knew, was willing and eager, but he had helped me at jobs before and his usefulness was impaired by the fact that his hands were always filled with his smoking items and he kept dropping things.

I got down on my knees behind the animal with the feeling that I was on my own. And as soon as I cradled the mass in my arms the conviction flooded through me that this was going to be the same as all the others. The very idea of this lot going back whence it came was ridiculous and the impression was reinforced as I began to push. Nothing happened.

I had sedated the sow heavily and she wasn't straining much against me; it was just that the thing was so huge. By a supreme effort I managed to feed a few inches back into the vaginal opening but as soon as I relaxed it popped quietly out again. My strongest instinct was to call the whole thing off without delay; the end result would be the same and anyway I wasn't feeling very strong. In fact my whole being was permeated by the leaden-armed pervading weakness one feels when forced to work in the small hours.

I would try just once more. Lying flat, my naked chest

against the cold concrete I fought with the thing till my eyes popped and my breath gave out, but it had not the slightest effect and it made my mind up; I had to tell him.

Rolling over on my back I looked up at him, panting, waiting till I had the wind to speak. I would say, 'Lord Hulton, we are really wasting our time here. This is an impossible case. I am going back home now and I'll ring the slaughterhouse first thing in the morning.' The prospect of escape was beguiling; I might even be able to crawl in beside Helen for an hour. But as my mouth framed the words the·little man looked down at me appealingly as though he knew what I was going to say. He tried to smile but darted anxious glances at me, at the pig and back again. From the other end of the animal a soft uncomplaining grunt reminded me that I wasn't the only one involved.

I didn't say anything. I turned back on to my chest, braced my feet against the wall of the pen and began again. I don't know how long I lay there, pushing, relaxing, pushing again as I gasped and groaned and the sweat ran steadily down my back. The peer was silent but I knew he was following my progress intently because every now and then I had to brush matches from the surface of the uterus.

Then for no particular reason the heap of flesh in my arms felt suddenly smaller. I glared desperately at the thing. There was no doubt about it, it was only half the size. I had to take a breather and a hoarse croak escaped me.

'God! I think it's going back!'

I must have startled Lord Hulton in mid fill because I heard a stifled 'What . . . what . . . oh I say, how absolutely splendid!' and a fragrant shower of tobacco cascaded from above.

This was it, then. Summoning the last of my energy for one big effort I blew half an ounce or so of Redbreast Flake from the uterine mucosa and heaved forward. And, miraculously, there was little resistance and I stared in disbelief as the great organ disappeared gloriously and wonderfully from sight. I was right behind it with my arm, probing frantically away up to the shoulder as I rotated my wrist again and again till both uterine cornua were fully involuted. When I was certain beyond doubt that everything was back in place I lay there for a few moments, my arm still deep inside the sow, my forehead resting on the floor. Dimly, through the mist of exhaustion I heard Lord Hulton's cries.

'Stout fella! Dash it, how marvellous! Oh stout fella!' He was almost dancing with joy.

One last terror assailed me. What if it came out again? Quickly I seized needle and thread and began to insert a few sutures in the vulva.

'Here, hold this!' I barked, giving him the scissors.

Stitching with the help of Lord Hulton wasn't easy. I kept pushing needle or scissors into his hands then demanding them back peremptorily, and it caused a certain amount of panic. Twice he passed me his pipe to cut the ends of my suture and on one occasion I found myself trying in the dim light to thread the silk through his reaming tool. His lordship suffered too, in his turn, because I heard the occasional stifled oath as he impaled a finger on the needle.

But at last it was done. I rose wearily to my feet and leaned against the wall, my mouth hanging open, sweat trickling into my eyes. The little man's eyes were full of concern as they roved over my limply hanging arms and the caked blood and filth on my chest.

'Herriot, my dear old chap, you're all in! And you'll catch pneumonia or something if you stand around half naked. You need a hot drink. Tell you what – get yourself cleaned up and dressed and I'll run down to the house for something.' He scurried swiftly away.

My aching muscles were slow to obey as I soaped and towelled myself and pulled on my shirt. Fastening my watch round my wrist I saw that it was after seven and I could hear the farm men clattering in the yard outside as they began their morning tasks.

I was buttoning my jacket when the little peer returned. He bore a tray with a pint mug of steaming coffee and two thick slices of bread and honey. He placed it on a bale of straw and pulled up an upturned bucket as a chair before hopping on to a meal bin where he sat like a pixie on a toadstool with his arms around his knees, regarding me with keen anticipation.

'The servants are still abed, old chap,' he said. 'So I made this little bite for you myself.'

I sank on to the bucket and took a long pull at the coffee. It was black and scalding with a kick like a Galloway bullock and it spread like fire through my tired frame. Then I bit into the first slice of bread; home made, plastered thickly with farm butter and topped by a lavish layer of heather honey from the long row of hives I had often seen on the edge of the moor above. I closed my eyes in reverence as I chewed, then as I reached for the pint pot again I looked up at the small figure on the bin.

'May I say, sir, that this isn't a bite, it's a feast. It is all absolutely delicious.'

His face lit up with impish glee. 'Well, dash it . . . do you really think so? I'm so pleased. And you've done nobly, dear boy. Can't tell you how grateful I am.'

As I continued to eat ecstatically, feeling the strength ebbing back, he glanced uneasily into the pen.

'Herriot . . . those stitches. Don't like the look of them much. . . .'

'Oh yes,' I said. 'They're just a precaution. You can nick them out in a couple of days.'

'Splendid! But won't they leave a wound? We'd better put something on there.'

I paused in mid chew. Here it was again. He only needed his Propamidine to complete his happiness.

'Yes, old chap, we must apply some of that Prip . . . Prom . . . oh hell and blast, it's no good!' He threw back his head and bellowed, 'Charlie!'

The foreman appeared in the entrance, touching his cap. 'Morning, m'lord.'

'Morning, Charlie. See that this sow gets some of that wonderful cream on her. What the blazes d'you call it again?'

Charlie swallowed and squared his shoulders. 'Propopamide, m'lord.'

The little man threw his arms high in delight. 'Of course, of course! Propopamide! I wonder if I'll ever be able to get that word out?' He looked admiringly at his foreman. 'Charlie, you never fail – I don't know how you do it.'

Charlie bowed gravely in acknowledgement.

Lord Hulton turned to me. 'You'll let us have some more Propopamide, won't you, Herriot?'

'Certainly,' I replied. 'I think I have some in the car.'

Sitting there on the bucket amid the mixed aromas of pig and barley meal and coffee I could almost feel the waves of pleasure beating on me. His lordship was clearly enchanted by the whole business, Charlie was wearing the superior smile which always accompanied his demonstrations of lingual dexterity, and as for myself I was experiencing a mounting euphoria.

I could see into the pen and the sight was rewarding. The little pigs who had been sheltered in a large box during the operation were back with their mother, side by side in a long pink row as their tiny mouths enclosed the teats. The sow seemed to be letting her milk down, too, because there was no frantic scramble for position, just a rapt concentration.

She was a fine pedigree pig and instead of lying on the butcher's slab today she would be starting to bring up her family. As though reading my thoughts she gave a series of contented grunts and the old feeling began to bubble in me, the deep sense of fulfilment and satisfaction that comes from even the smallest triumph and makes our lives worth while.

And there was something else. A new thought stealing into my consciousness with a delicious fresh tingle about it. At this moment, who else in the length and breadth of Britain was eating a breakfast personally prepared and served by a marquis?

three

I am afraid of dentists.

I am particularly afraid of strange dentists, so before I went into the RAF I made sure my teeth were in order. Everybody told me they were very strict about the aircrew's teeth and I didn't want some unknown prodding around in my mouth. There had to be no holes anywhere or they would start to ache away up there in the sky, so they said.

So before my call-up I went to old Mr Grover in Darrowby and he painstakingly did all that was necessary. He was good at his job and was always gentle and careful and didn't strike the same terror into me as other dentists. All I felt when I went to his surgery was a dryness of the throat and a quivering at the knees, and providing I kept my eyes tightly shut all the time I managed to get through the visit fairly easily.

My fear of dentists dates back to my earliest experiences in the twenties. As a child I was taken to the dread Hector McDarroch in Glasgow and he did my dental work right up to my teens. Friends of my youth tell me that he inspired a similar lasting fear in them, too, and in fact there must be a whole generation of Glaswegians who feel the same.

Of course you couldn't blame Hector entirely. The equipment in those days was primitive and a visit to any dental practitioner was an ordeal. But Hector, with his booming laugh, was so large and overpowering that he made it worse. Actually he was a very nice man, cheerful and good-natured, but the other side of him blotted it all out.

The electric drill had not yet been invented or if it had, it hadn't reached Scotland, and Hector bored holes in teeth with a fearsome foot-operated machine. There was a great wheel driven by a leather belt and this powered the drill, and as you lay in the chair two things dominated the outlook; the wheel whirring by your ear and Hector's huge knee pistoning almost into your face as he pedalled furiously.

He came from the far north and at the Highland games he

used to array himself in kilt and sporran and throw cabers around like matchsticks. He was so big and strong that I always felt hopelessly trapped in that chair with his bulk over me and the wheel grinding and the pedal thumping. He didn't exactly put his foot on my chest but he had me all right.

And it didn't worry him when he got into the sensitive parts with his drill; my strangled cries were of no avail and he carried on remorselessly to the end. I had the impression that Hector thought it was cissy to feel pain, or maybe he was of the opinion that suffering was good for the soul.

Anyway, since those days I've had a marked preference for small frail soft-spoken dentists like Mr Grover. I like to feel that if it came to a stand-up fight I would have a good chance of victory and escape. Also, Mr Grover understood that people were afraid, and that helped. I remember him chuckling when he told me about the big farm men who came to have their teeth extracted. Many a time, he said, he had gone across the room for his instruments and turned back to find the chair empty.

I still don't enjoy going to the dentist but I have to admit that the modern men are wonderful. I hardly see mine when I go. Just a brief glimpse of a white coat then all is done from behind. Fingers come round, things go in and out of my mouth but even when I venture to open my eyes I see nothing.

Hector McDarroch, on the other hand, seemed to take a pleasure in showing off his grisly implements, filling the long-needled syringe right in front of my eyes and squirting the cocaine ceilingwards a few times before he started on me. And worse, before an extraction he used to clank about in a tin box, producing a series of hideous forceps and examining them, whistling softly, till he found the right one.

So with all this in mind, as I sat in a long queue of airmen for the preliminary examination, I was thankful I had been to Mr Grover for a complete check-up. A dentist stood by a chair at the end of the long room and he examined the young men in blue one by one before calling out his findings to an orderly at a desk.

I derived considerable entertainment from watching the expressions on the lads' faces when the call went out. 'Three fillings, two extractions!' 'Eight fillings!' Most of them looked stunned, some thunderstruck, others almost tearful. Now and again one would try to expostulate with the man in white but it was no good; nobody was listening. At times I could have laughed out loud. Mind you, I felt a bit mean at being amused, but after all they had only themselves to blame. If only they had shown my foresight they would have had nothing to worry about.

When my name was called I strolled across, humming a little tune, and dropped nonchalantly into the chair. It didn't take the man long. He poked his way swiftly along my teeth then rapped out, 'Five fillings and one extraction!'

I sat bolt upright and stared at him in amazement.

'But . . . but . . .' I began to yammer, 'I had a check up by my own . . .'

'Next, please,' murmured the dentist.

'But Mr Grover said . . .'

'Next man! Move along!' bawled the orderly, and as I shuffled away I gazed appealingly at the white-coated figure. But he was reciting a list of my premolars and incisors and showed no interest.

I was still trembling when I was handed the details of my fate.

'Report at Regent Lodge tomorrow morning for the extraction,' the WAAF girl said.

Tomorrow morning! By God, they didn't mess about! And what the heck did it all mean, anyway? My teeth were perfectly sound. There was only that one with the bit of enamel chipped off. Mr Grover had pointed it out and said it wouldn't give any trouble. It was the tooth that held my pipe – surely it couldn't be that one.

But there came the disquieting thought that my opinion didn't matter. When my feeble protests were ignored back there it hit me for the first time that I wasn't a civilian any more.

Next morning the din from the dustbin lids had hardly

subsided when the grim realization drove into my brain. I was going to have a tooth out today! And very soon too. I passed the intervening hours in growing apprehension; morning parade, the march through the darkness to breakfast. The dried egg and fried bread were less attractive than ever and the grey day had hardly got under way before I was approaching the forbidding façade of Regent Lodge.

As I climbed the steps my palms began to sweat. I didn't like having my teeth drilled but extractions were infinitely worse. Something in me recoiled from the idea of having a part of myself torn away by force, even if it didn't hurt. But of course, I told myself as I walked along an echoing corridor, it never did hurt nowadays. Just a little prick, then nothing.

I was nurturing this comforting thought when I turned into a large assembly room with numbered doors leading from it. About thirty airmen sat around wearing a variety of expressions from sickly smiles to tough bravado. A chilling smell of antiseptic hung on the air. I chose a chair and settled down to wait. I had been in the armed forces long enough to know that you waited a long time for everything and I saw no reason why a dental appointment should be any different.

As I sat down the man on my left gave me a brief nod. He was fat, and greasy black hair fell over his pimpled brow. Though engrossed in picking his teeth with a match he gave me a long appraising stare before addressing me in rich cockney.

'What room you goin' in, mate?'

I looked at my card. 'Room four.'

'Blimey, mate, you've 'ad it!' He removed his matchstick and grinned wolfishly.

'Had it . . . ? What do you mean?'

'Well, haven't you 'eard? That's The Butcher in there.'

'The . . . The . . . Butcher?' I quavered.

'Yeh, that's what they call the dental officer in there.' He gave an expansive smile. 'He's a right killer, that bloke, I'll tell yer.'

I swallowed. 'Butcher . . . ? Killer . . . ? Oh come on. They'll all be the same, I'm sure.'

'Don't you believe it, mate. There's good an' there's bad, and that bloke's pure murder. It shouldn't be allowed.'

'How do you know, anyway?'

He waved an airy hand. 'Oh I've been 'ere a few times and I've heard some bleedin' awful screams comin' out of that room. Spoken to some of the chaps afterwards, too. They all call 'im The Butcher.'

I rubbed my hands on the rough blue of my trousers. 'Oh you hear these tales. I'm sure they're exaggerated'

'Well, you'll find out, mate.' He resumed his tooth picking. 'But don't say I didn't tell you.'

He went on about various things but I only half heard him. His name, it seemed, was Simkin, and he was not an aircrew cadet like the rest of us but a regular and a member of the groundstaff; he worked in the kitchens. He spoke scornfully of us raw recruits and pointed out that we would have to 'get some service in' before we were fit to associate with the real members of the Royal Air Force. I noticed, however, that despite his own years of allegiance he was still an AC2 like myself.

Almost an hour passed with my heart thumping every time the door of number four opened. I had to admit that the young men leaving that room all looked a bit shattered and one almost reeled out, holding his mouth with both hands.

'Cor! Look at that poor bugger!' Simkin drawled with ill-concealed satisfaction. 'Strike me! He's been through it, poor bleeder. I'm glad I'm not in your shoes. mate.'

I could feel the tension mounting in me. 'What room are you going into, anyway?' I asked.

He did a bit of deep exploration with his match. 'Room two, mate. I've been in there before. He's a grand bloke, one of the best. Never 'urts you.'

'Well you're lucky, aren't you?'

'Not lucky, mate.' He paused and stabbed his match at me. 'I know my way around, that's all. There's ways and means.' He allowed one eyelid to drop briefly.

The conversation was abruptly terminated as the dread door opened and a WAAF came out.

'AC2 Herriot!' she called.

I got up on shaking limbs and took a deep breath. As I set off I had a fleeting glimpse of the leer of pure delight on Simkin's face. He was really enjoying himself.

As I passed the portals my feeling of doom increased. The Butcher was another Hector McDarroch; about six feet two with rugby forward shoulders bulging his white coat. My flesh crept as he unleashed a hearty laugh and motioned me towards the chair.

As I sat down I decided to have one last try.

'Is this the tooth?' I asked, tapping the only possible suspect.

'It is indeed!' boomed The Butcher. 'That's the one.'

'Ah well,' I said with a light laugh. 'I'm sure I can explain. There's been some mistake. . . .'

'Yes . . . yes. . . .' he murmured, filling the syringe before my eyes and sending a few playful spurts into the air.

'There's just a bit of enamel off it, and Mr Grover said . . .'

The WAAF suddenly wound the chair back and I found myself in the semi-prone position with the white bulk looming over me.

'You see,' I gasped desperately. 'I need that tooth. It's the one that holds my . . .'

A strong finger was on my gum and I felt the needle going in. I resigned myself to my fate.

When he had inserted the local the big man put the syringe down. 'We'll just give that a minute or two,' he said, and left the room.

As soon as the door closed behind him the WAAF tiptoed over to me.

'This feller's loopy!' she whispered.

Half lying, I stared at her.

'Loopy . . . ? What d'you mean?'

'Crackers! Round the bend! No idea how to pull teeth!'

'But . . . but . . . he's a dentist isn't he . . . ?'

She pulled a wry face, 'Thinks he is! But he hasn't a clue!'

I had no time to explore this cheering information further because the door opened and the big man returned.

He seized a horrible pair of forceps and I closed my eyes as he started flexing his muscles.

I must admit I felt nothing. I knew he was twisting and tugging away up there but the local had mercifully done its job. I was telling myself that it would soon be over when I heard a sharp crack.

I opened my eyes. The Butcher was gazing disappointedly at my broken-off tooth in his forceps. The root was still in my gum.

Behind him the WAAF gave me a long 'I told you so' nod. She was a pretty little thing, but I fear the libido of the young men she encountered in here would be at a low ebb.

'Oh!' The Butcher grunted and began to rummage in a metal box. It took me right to the McDarroch days as he fished out one forceps after another, opened and shut them a few times then tried them on me.

But it was of no avail, and as the time passed I was the un-willing witness of the gradual transition from heartiness to silence, then to something like panic. The man was clearly whacked. He had no idea how to shift that root.

He must have been gouging for half an hour when an idea seemed to strike him. Pushing all the forceps to one side he almost ran from the room and reappeared shortly with a tray on which reposed a long chisel and a metal mallet.

At a sign from him the WAAF wound the chair back till I was completely horizontal. Seemingly familiar with the routine, she cradled my head in her arms in a practised manner and stood waiting.

This couldn't be true, I thought, as the man inserted the chisel into my mouth and poised the mallet; but all doubts were erased as the metal rod thudded against the remnants of my tooth and my head in turn shot back into the little WAAF's bosom. And that was how it went on. I lost count of time as The Butcher banged away and the girl hung on grimly to my jerking skull.

The thought uppermost in my mind was that I had always wondered how young horses felt when I knocked wolf teeth out of them. Now I knew.

When it finally stopped I opened my eyes, and though by this time I was prepared for anything I still felt slightly surprised to see The Butcher threading a needle with a length of suture silk. He was sweating and looking just a little desperate as he bent over yet again.

'Just a couple of stitches,' he muttered hoarsely, and I closed my eyes again.

When I left the chair I felt very strange indeed. The assault on my cranium had made me dizzy and the sensation of the long ends of the stitches tickling my tongue was distinctly odd. I'm sure that when I came out of the room I was staggering, and instinctively I pawed at my mouth.

The first man I saw was Simkin. He was where I had left him but he looked different as he beckoned excitedly to me. I went over and he caught at my tunic with one hand.

'What d'yer think, mate?' he gasped. 'They've changed me round and I've got to go into room four.' He gulped. 'You looked bloody awful comin' out there. What was it like?'

I looked at him Maybe there was going to be a gleam of light this morning. I sank into the chair next to him and groaned.

'By God, you weren't kidding! I've never met anybody like that – he's half killed me. They don't call him The Butcher for nothing!'

'Why . . . what . . . what did 'e do?'

'Nothing much. Just knocked my tooth out with a hammer and chisel, that's all.'

'Garn! You're 'avin' me on!' Simkin made a ghastly attempt to smile.

'Word of honour,' I said. 'Anyway, there's the tray coming out now. Look for yourself.'

He stared at the WAAF carrying the dreadful implements and turned very pale.

'Oh blimey! What . . . what else did 'e do?'

I held my jaw for a moment. 'Well he did something I've never seen before. He made such a great hole in my gum that he had to stitch me up afterwards.'

Simkin shook his head violently. 'Naow, I'm not 'avin' that! I don't believe yer!'

'All right,' I said. 'What do you think of this?'

I leaned forward, put my thumb under my lip and jerked it up to give him a close-up view of the long gash and the trailing blood-stained ends of the stitches.

He shrank away from me, lips trembling, eyes wide.

'Gawd!' he moaned. 'Oh Gawd . . . !'

It was unfortunate that the WAAF chose that particular moment to call out 'AC2 Simkin' piercingly from the doorway, because the poor fellow leaped as though a powerful electric current had passed through him. Then, head down, he trailed across the room. At the door he turned and gave me a last despairing look and I saw him no more.

This experience deepened my dread of the five fillings which awaited me. But I needn't have worried; they were trivial things and were efficiently and painlessly dealt with by RAF dentists very different from The Butcher.

And yet, many years after the war had ended, the man from room four stretched out a long arm from the past and touched me on the shoulder. I began to feel something sharp coming through the roof of my mouth and went to Mr Grover, who X-rayed me and showed me a pretty picture of that fateful root still there despite the hammer and chisel. He extracted it and the saga was ended.

The Butcher remained a vivid memory because, apart from my ordeal, I was constantly reminded of him by the dangerous wobbling of my pipe at the edge of that needless gap in my mouth. But I did have a small solace. I finished my visit to room four with a parting shaft which gave me a little comfort. As I tottered away I paused and addressed the big man's back as he prepared for his next victim.

'By the way,' I said. 'I've knocked out a lot of teeth just like you did there.'

He turned and stared at me. 'Really? Are you a dentist?'

'No,' I replied over my shoulder as I left. 'I'm a vet!'

four

I like women better than men.

Mind you, I have nothing against men – after all, I am one myself – but in the RAF there were too many of them. Literally thousands, jostling, shouting, swearing; you couldn't get away from them. Some of them became my friends and have remained so until the present day, but the sheer earthy mass of them made me realize how my few months of married life had changed me.

Women are gentler, softer, cleaner, altogether nicer things and I, who always considered myself one of the boys, had come to the surprising conclusion that the companion I wanted most was a woman.

My impression that I had been hurled into a coarser world was heightened at the beginning of each day, particularly one morning when I was on fire picket duty and had the sadistic pleasure of rattling the dustbin lids and shouting 'Wakey-wakey!' along the corridors. It wasn't the cursing and the obscene remarks which struck deepest, it was the extraordinary abdominal noises issuing from the dark rooms. They reminded me of my patient, Cedric, and in an instant I was back in Darrowby answering the telephone.

The voice at the other end was oddly hesitant.

'Mr Herriot . . . I should be grateful if you would come and see my dog.' It was a woman, obviously upper class.

'Certainly. What's the trouble?'

'Well . . . he . . . er . . . he seems to suffer from . . . a certain amount of flatus.'

'I beg your pardon?'

There was a long pause. 'He has . . . excessive flatus.'

'In what way, exactly?'

'Well . . . I suppose you'd describe it as . . . windiness.' The voice had begun to tremble.

I thought I could see a gleam of light. 'You mean his stomach . . . ?'

'No, not his stomach. He passes ... er ... a considerable quantity of ... wind from his ... his ...' A note of desperation had crept in.

'Ah, yes!' All became suddenly clear. 'I quite understand. But that doesn't sound very serious. Is he ill?'

'No, he's very fit in other ways.'

'Well then, do you think it's necessary for me to see him?'

'Oh yes, indeed, Mr Herriot. I wish you would come as soon as possible. It has become quite ... quite a problem.'

'All right,' I said. 'I'll look in this morning. Can I have your name and address, please?'

'It's Mrs Rumney, The Laurels.'

The Laurels was a very nice house on the edge of the town standing back from the road in a large garden. Mrs Rumney herself let me in and I felt a shock of surprise at my first sight of her. It wasn't just that she was strikingly beautiful; there was an unworldly air about her. She would be around forty but had the appearance of a heroine in a Victorian novel – tall, willowy, ethereal. And I could understand immediately her hesitation on the phone. Everything about her suggested fastidiousness and delicacy.

'Cedric is in the kitchen,' she said. 'I'll take you through.'

I had another surprise when I saw Cedric. An enormous boxer hurled himself on me in delight, clawing at my chest with the biggest, horniest feet I had seen for a long time. I tried to fight him off but he kept at me, panting ecstatically into my face and wagging his entire rear end.

'Sit down, boy!' the lady said sharply, then, as Cedric took absolutely no notice, she turned to me nervously. 'He's so friendly.'

'Yes,' I said breathlessly, 'I can see that.' I finally managed to push the huge animal away and backed into a corner for safety. 'How often does this ... excessive flatus occur?'

As if in reply an almost palpable sulphurous wave arose from the dog and eddied around me. It appeared that the excitement of seeing me had activated Cedric's weakness. I was up against the wall and unable to obey my first instinct to run for cover so I held my hand over my face for a few moments before speaking.

'Is that what you meant?'

Mrs Rumney waved a lace handkerchief under her nose and the faintest flush crept into the pallor of her cheeks.

'Yes,' she replied almost inaudibly. 'Yes . . . that is it.'

'Oh well,' I said briskly. 'There's nothing to worry about. Let's go into the other room and we'll have a word about his diet and a few other things.'

It turned out that Cedric was getting rather a lot of meat and I drew up a little chart cutting down the protein and adding extra carbohydrates. I prescribed a kaolin antacid mixture to be given night and morning and left the house in a confident frame of mind.

It was one of those trivial things and I had entirely forgotten it when Mrs Rumney phoned again.

'I'm afraid Cedric is no better, Mr Herriot.'

'Oh I'm sorry to hear that. He's still . . . er . . . still . . . yes . . . yes . . .' I spent a few moments in thought. 'I tell you what – I don't think I can do any more by seeing him at the moment, but I think you should cut out his meat completely for a week or two. Keep him on biscuits and brown bread rusked in the oven. Try him with that and vegetables and I'll give you some powder to mix in his food. Perhaps you'd call round for it.'

The powder was a pretty strong absorbent mixture and I felt sure it would do the trick, but a week later Mrs Rumney was on the phone again.

'There's absolutely no improvement, Mr Herriot.' The tremble was back in her voice. 'I . . . I do wish you'd come and see him again.'

I couldn't see much point in viewing this perfectly healthy animal again but I promised to call. I had a busy day and it was after six o'clock before I got round to The Laurels. There were several cars in the drive and when I went into the house I saw that Mrs Rumney had a few people in for drinks; people like herself – upper class and of obvious refinement. In fact I felt rather a lout in my working clothes among the elegant gathering.

Mrs Rumney was about to lead me through to the kitchen when the door burst open and Cedric bounded delightedly into the midst of the company. Within seconds an aesthetic-looking gentleman was frantically beating off the attack as the great feet ripped down his waistcoat. He got away at the cost of a couple of buttons and the boxer turned his attention to one of the ladies. She was in imminent danger of losing her dress when I pulled the dog off her.

Pandemonium broke out in the graceful room. The hostess's plaintive appeals rang out above the cries of alarm as the big dog charged around, but very soon I realized that a more insidious element had crept into the situation. The atmosphere in the room became rapidly charged with an unmistakable effluvium and it was clear that Cedric's unfortunate malady had reasserted itself.

I did my best to shepherd the animal out of the room but he didn't seem to know the meaning of obedience and I chased him in vain. And as the embarrassing minutes ticked away I began to realize for the first time the enormity of the problem which confronted Mrs Rumney. Most dogs break wind occasionally but Cedric was different; he did it all the time. And while his silent emanations were perhaps more treacherous there was no doubt that the audible ones were painfully distressing in a company like this.

Cedric made it worse, because at each rasping expulsion he would look round enquiringly at his back end then gambol about the room as though the fugitive zephyr was clearly visible to him and he was determined to corner it.

It seemed a year before I got him out of there. Mrs Rumney held the door wide as I finally managed to steer him towards it but the big dog wasn't finished yet. On his way out he cocked a leg swiftly and directed a powerful jet against an immaculate trouser leg.

After that night I threw myself into the struggle on Mrs Rumney's behalf. I felt she desperately needed my help, and I made frequent visits and tried innumerable remedies. I consulted my colleague Siegfried on the problem and he suggested a diet of charcoal biscuits. Cedric ate them in vast quantities and with evident enjoyment but they, like everything else, made not the slightest difference to his condition.

And all the time I pondered upon the enigma of Mrs Rumney. She had lived in Darrowby for several years but the townsfolk knew little about her. It was a matter of debate whether she was a widow or separated from her husband. But I was not interested in such things; the biggest mystery to me was how she ever got involved with a dog like Cedric.

It was difficult to think of any animal less suited to her personality. Apart from his regrettable affliction he was in every way the opposite to herself; a great thick-headed, rumbustious extrovert totally out of place in her gracious menage. I never did find out how they came together but on my visits I found that Cedric had one admirer at least.

He was Con Fenton, a retired farm worker who did a bit of jobbing gardening and spent an average of three days a week at The Laurels. The boxer romped down the drive after me as I was leaving and the old man looked at him with undisguised admiration.

'By gaw,' he said. 'He's a fine dog, is that!'

'Yes, he is, Con, he's a good chap, really.' And I meant it. You couldn't help liking Cedric when you got to know him. He was utterly amiable and without vice and he gave off a constant aura not merely of noxious vapours but of bonhomie. When he tore off people's buttons or sprinkled their trousers he did it in a spirit of the purest amity.

'Just look at them limbs!' breathed Con, staring rapturously at the dog's muscular thighs. 'By heck, 'e can jump ower that gate as if it weren't there. He's what ah call a dog!'

As he spoke it struck me that Cedric would be likely to appeal to him because he was very like the boxer himself; not over-burdened with brains, built like an ox with powerful shoulders and a big constantly-grinning face – they were two of a kind.

'Aye, ah allus likes it when t'missus lets him out in t'garden,' Con went on. He always spoke in a peculiar snuffling manner. 'He's grand company.'

I looked at him narrowly. No, he wouldn't be likely to notice Cedric's complaint since he always saw him out of doors.

On my way back to the surgery I brooded on the fact that I was achieving absolutely nothing with my treatment. And though it seemed ridiculous to worry about a case like this, there was no doubt the thing had begun to prey on my mind. In fact I began to transmit my anxieties to Siegfried. As I got out of the car he was coming down the steps of Skeldale House and he put a hand on my arm.

'You've been to The Laurels, James? Tell me,' he enquired solicitously, 'how is your farting boxer today?'

'Still at it, I'm afraid,' I replied, and my colleague shook his head in commiseration.

We were both defeated. Maybe if chlorophyll tablets had been available in those days they might have helped but as it was I had tried everything. It seemed certain that nothing would alter the situation. And it wouldn't have been so bad if the owner had been anybody else but Mrs Rumney; I found that even discussing the thing with her had become almost unbearable.

Siegfried's student brother Tristan didn't help, either. When seeing practice he was very selective in the cases he wished to observe, but he was immediately attracted to Cedric's symptoms and insisted on coming with me on one occasion. I never took him again because as we went in the big dog bounded from his mistress' side and produced a particularly sonorous blast as if in greeting.

Tristan immediately threw out a hand in a dramatic gesture and declaimed: 'Speak on, sweet lips that never told a lie!' That was his only visit. I had enough trouble without that.

I didn't know it at the time but a greater blow awaited me. A few days later Mrs Rumney was on the phone again.

'Mr Herriot, a friend of mine has such a sweet little Boxer bitch. She wants to bring her along to be mated with Cedric.'

'Eh?'

'She wants to mate her bitch with my dog.'

'With Cedric . . . ?' I clutched at the edge of the desk. It couldn't be true! 'And . . . and are you agreeable?'

'Yes, of course.'

I shook my head to dispel the feeling of unreality. I found it incomprehensible that anyone should want to reproduce Cedric, and as I gaped into the receiver a frightening vision floated before me of eight little Cedrics all with his complaint. But of course such a thing wasn't hereditary. I took a grip of myself and cleared my throat.

'Very well, then, Mrs Rumney, you'd better go ahead.'

There was a pause. 'But Mr Herriot, I want you to supervise the mating.'

'Oh really, I don't think that's necessary.' I dug my nails into my palm. 'I think you'll be all right without me.'

'Oh but I would be much happier if you were there. Please come,' she said appealingly.

Instead of emitting a long-drawn groan I took a deep breath.

'Right,' I said. 'I'll be along in the morning.'

All that evening I was obsessed by a feeling of dread. Another acutely embarrassing session was in store with this exquisite woman. Why was it I always had to share things like this with her? And I really feared the worst. Even the daftest dog, when confronted with a bitch in heat, knows instinctively how to proceed, but with a really ivory-skulled animal like Cedric I wondered. . . .

And next morning all my fears were realized. The bitch, Trudy, was a trim little creature and showed every sign of willingness to cooperate. Cedric, on the other hand, though obviously delighted to meet her, gave no hint of doing his part. After sniffing her over, he danced around her a few times, goofy-faced, tongue lolling. Then he had a roll on the lawn before charging at her and coming to a full stop, big feet outsplayed, head down, ready to play. I sighed. It was as I thought. The big chump didn't know what to do.

This pantomime went on for some time and, inevitably, the emotional strain brought on a resurgence of his symptoms. Frequently he paused to inspect his tail as though he had never heard noises like that before.

He varied his dancing routine with occasional headlong gallops round the lawn and it was after he had done about ten successive laps that he seemed to decide he ought to do something about the bitch. I held my breath as he approached her but unfortunately he chose the wrong end to commence operations. Trudy had put up with his nonsense with great patience but when she found him busily working away in the region of her left ear it was too much. With a shrill yelp she nipped him in the hind leg and he shot away in alarm.

After that whenever he came near she warned him off with bared teeth. Clearly she was disenchanted with her bridegroom and I couldn't blame her.

'I think she's had enough, Mrs Rumney,' I said.

I certainly had had enough and so had the poor lady, judging by her slight breathlessness, flushed cheeks and waving handkerchief.

'Yes . . . yes . . . I suppose you're right,' she replied.

So Trudy was taken home and that was the end of Cedric's career as a stud dog.

This last episode decided me. I had to have a talk with Mrs Rumney and a few days later I called in at The Laurels.

'Maybe you'll think it's none of my business,' I said. 'But I honestly don't think Cedric is the dog for you. In fact he's so wrong for you that he is upsetting your life.'

Mrs Rumney's eyes widened. 'Well . . . he is a problem in some ways . . . but what do you suggest?'

'I think you should get another dog in his place. Maybe a poodle or a corgi – something smaller, something you could control.'

'But Mr Herriot, I couldn't possibly have Cedric put down.' Her eyes filled quickly with tears. 'I really am fond of him despite his . . . despite everything.'

'No, no, of course not!' I said. 'I like him too. He has no malice in him. But I think I have a good idea. Why not let Con Fenton have him?'

'Con . . . ?'

'Yes, he admires Cedric tremendously and the big fellow would have a good life with the old man. He has a couple of fields behind his cottage and keeps a few beasts. Cedric could run to his heart's content out there and Con would be able to bring him along when he does the garden. You'd still see him three times a week.'

Mrs Rumney looked at me in silence for a few moments and I saw in her face the dawning of relief and hope.

'You know, Mr Herriot, I think that could work very well. But are you sure Con would take him?'

'I'd like to bet on it. An old bachelor like him must be lonely. There's only one thing worries me. Normally they only meet outside and I wonder how it would be when they were indoors and Cedric started to ... when the old trouble ... '

'Oh, I think that would be all right,' Mrs Rumney broke in quickly. 'When I go on holiday Con always takes him for a week or two and he has never mentioned any ... anything unusual ... in that way.'

I got up to go. 'Well, that's fine. I should put it to the old man right away.'

Mrs Rumney rang within a few days. Con had jumped at the chance of taking Cedric and the pair had apparently settled in happily together. She had also taken my advice and acquired a poodle puppy.

I didn't see the new dog till it was nearly six months old and its mistress asked me to call to treat it for a slight attack of eczema. As I sat in the graceful room looking at Mrs Rumney, cool, poised, tranquil, with the little white creature resting on her knee I couldn't help feeling how right and fitting the whole scene was. The lush carpet, the trailing velvet curtains, the fragile tables with their load of expensive china and framed miniatures. It was no place for Cedric.

Con Fenton's cottage was less than half a mile away and on my way back to the surgery, on an impulse I pulled up at the door. The old man answered my knock and his big face split into a delighted grin when he saw me.

'Come in, young man!' he cried in his strange snuffly voice. 'I'm right glad to see tha!'

I had hardly stepped into the tiny living room when a hairy form hurled itself upon me. Cedric hadn't changed a bit and I had to battle my way to the broken armchair by the fireside.

Con settled down opposite and when the boxer leaped to lick his face he clumped him companionably on the head with his fist.

'Siddown, ye great daft bugger,' he murmured with affection. Cedric sank happily on to the tattered hearthrug at his feet and gazed up adoringly at his new master.

'Well, Mr Herriot,' Con went on as he cut up some villainous-looking plug tobacco and began to stuff it into his pipe. 'I'm right grateful to ye for gettin' me this grand dog. By gaw, he's a topper and ah wouldn't sell 'im for any money. No man could ask for a better friend.'

'Well that's great, Con,' I said. 'And I can see that the big chap is really happy here.'

The old man ignited his pipe and a cloud of acrid smoke rose to the low, blackened beams. 'Aye, he's 'ardly ever inside. A gurt strong dog like 'im wants to work 'is energy off, like.'

But just at that moment Cedric was obviously working something else off because the familiar pungency rose from him even above the billowings from the pipe. Con seemed oblivious of it but in the enclosed space I found it overpowering.

'Ah well,' I gasped. 'I just looked in for a moment to see how you were getting on together. I must be on my way.' I rose hurriedly and stumbled towards the door but the redolence followed me in a wave. As I passed the table with the remains of the old man's meal I saw what seemed to be the only form of ornament in the cottage, a cracked vase holding a magnificent bouquet of carnations. It was a way of escape and I buried my nose in their fragrance.

Con watched me approvingly. 'Aye, they're lovely flowers, aren't they? T'missus at Laurels lets me bring 'ome what I want and I reckon them carnations is me favourite.'

'Yes, they're a credit to you.' I still kept my nose among the blooms.

'There's only one thing,' the old man said pensively. 'Ah don't get t'full benefit of 'em.'

'How's that, Con?'

He pulled at his pipe a couple of times. 'Well, you can hear ah speak a bit funny, like?'

'No . . . no . . . not really.'

'Oh aye, ye know ah do. I've been like it since I were a lad. I 'ad a operation for adenoids and summat went wrong.'

'Oh, I'm sorry to hear that,' I said.

'Well, it's nowt serious, but it's left me lackin' in one way.'

'You mean . . . ?' A light was beginning to dawn in my mind, an elucidation of how man and dog had found each other, of why their relationship was so perfect, of the certainty of their happy future together. It seemed like fate.

'Aye,' the old man went on sadly. 'I 'ave no sense of smell.'

five

I think it was when I saw the London policeman wagging a finger at a scowling urchin that I thought of Wesley Binks and the time he put the firework through the surgery letter box.

It was what they used to call a 'banger' and it exploded at my feet as I hurried along the dark passage in answer to the door bell's ring, making me leap into the air in terror.

I threw open the front door and looked into the street. It was empty, but at the corner where the lamplight was reflected in Robson's shop window I had a brief impression of a fleeing form and a faint echo of laughter. I couldn't do anything about it but I knew Wes was out there somewhere.

Wearily I trailed back into the house. Why did this lad persecute me? What could a ten-year-old boy possibly have against me? I had never done him any harm, yet I seemed to be the object of a deliberate campaign.

Or maybe it wasn't personal. It could be that he felt I

represented authority or the establishment in some way, or perhaps I was just convenient.

I was certainly the ideal subject for his little tricks of ringing the door bell and running away, because I dared not ignore the summons in case it might be a client, and also the consulting and operating rooms were such a long way from the front of the house. Sometimes I was dragged down from our bed-sitter under the tiles. Every trip to the door was an expedition and it was acutely exasperating to arrive there and see only a little figure in the distance dancing about and grimacing at me.

He varied this routine by pushing rubbish through the letter box, pulling the flowers from the tiny strip of garden we tried to cultivate between the flagstones and chalking rude messages on my car.

I knew I wasn't the only victim because I had heard complaints from others; the fruiterer who saw his apples disappear from the box in front of the shop, the grocer who unwillingly supplied him with free biscuits.

He was the town naughty boy all right, and it was incongruous that he should have been named Wesley. There was not the slightest sign in his behaviour of any strict Methodist upbringing. In fact I knew nothing of his family life – only that he came from the poorest part of the town, a row of 'yards' containing tumbledown cottages, some of them evacuated because of their condition.

I often saw him wandering about in the fields and lanes or fishing in quiet reaches of the river when he should have been in school. When he spotted me on these occasions he invariably called out some mocking remark and if he happened to be with some of his cronies they all joined in the laughter at my expense. It was annoying but I used to tell myself that there was nothing personal in it. I was an adult and that was enough to make me a target.

Wes's greatest triumph was undoubtedly the time he removed the grating from the coal cellar outside Skeldale House. It was on the left of the front steps and underneath it was a steep ramp down which the coalmen tipped their bags.

I don't know whether it was inspired intuition but he pinched the grating on the day of the Darrowby Gala. The festivities started with a parade through the town led by the Houlton Silver Band and as I looked down from the windows of our bed-sitter I could see them all gathering in the street below.

'Look, Helen,' I said. 'They must be starting the march from Trengate. Everybody I know seems to be down there.'

Helen leaned over my shoulder and gazed at the long lines of boy scouts, girl guides, ex-servicemen, with half the population of the town packed on the pavements, watching. 'Yes, it's quite a sight, isn't it? Let's go down and see them move off.'

We trotted down the long flights of stairs and I followed her out through the front door. And as I appeared in the entrance I was suddenly conscious that I was the centre of attention. The citizens on the pavements, waiting patiently for the parade to start, had something else to look at now. The little brownies and wolf cubs waved at me from their ranks and there were nods and smiles from the people across the road and on all sides.

I could divine their thoughts. 'There's t'young vitnery coming out of his house. Not long married, too. That's his missus next to him.'

A feeling of wellbeing rose in me. I don't know whether other newly married men feel the same, but in those early days I was aware of a calm satisfaction and fulfilment. And I was proud to be the 'vitnery' and part of the life of the town. There was my plate on the wall beside me, a symbol of my solid importance. I was a man of substance now, I had arrived.

Looking around me, I acknowledged the greeting with a few dignified little smiles, raising a gracious hand now and then rather like a royal personage on view. Then I noticed that Helen hadn't much room by my side, so I stepped to the left to where the grating should have been and slid gracefully down into the cellar.

It would be a dramatic touch to say I disappeared from

view; in fact I wish I had, because I would have stayed down there and avoided further embarrassment. But as it was I travelled only so far down the ramp and stuck there with my head and shoulders protruding into the street.

My little exhibition caused a sensation among the spectators. Nothing in the Gala parade could compete with this. One or two of the surrounding faces expressed alarm but loud laughter was the general response. The adults were almost holding each other up but the little brownies and wolf cubs made my most appreciative audience, breaking their ranks and staggering about helplessly in the roadway while their leaders tried to restore order.

I caused chaos, too, in the Houlton Silver Band, who were hoisting their instruments prior to marching off. If they had any ideas about bursting into tune they had to abandon them temporarily because I don't think any of them had breath to blow.

It was, in fact, two of the bandsmen who extricated me by linking their hands under my armpits. My wife was of no service at all in the crisis and I could only look up at her reproachfully as she leaned against the doorpost dabbing at her eyes.

It all became clear to me when I reached street level. I was flicking the coal dust from my trousers and trying to look unconcerned when I saw Wesley Binks doubled up with mirth, pointing triumphantly at me and at the hole over the cellar. He was quite near, jostling among the spectators, and I had my first close look at the wild-eyed little goblin who had plagued me. I may have made an unconscious movement towards him because he gave me a last malevolent grin and disappeared into the crowd.

Later I asked Helen about him. She could only tell me that Wesley's father had left home when he was about six years old, that his mother had remarried and the boy now lived with her and his stepfather.

Strangely, I had another opportunity to study him quite soon afterwards. It was about a week later and my feathers were still a little ruffled after the grating incident when I saw him sitting all alone in the waiting room. Alone, that is, except for a skinny black dog in his lap.

I could hardly believe it. I had often rehearsed the choice phrases which I would use on this very occasion but the sight of the animal restrained me; if he had come to consult me professionally I could hardly start pitching into him right away. Maybe later.

I pulled on a white coat and went in.

'Well, what can I do for you?' I asked coldly.

The boy stood up and his expression of mixed defiance and desperation showed that it had cost him something to enter this house.

'Summat matter wi' me dog,' he muttered.

'Right, bring him through.' I led the way along the passage to the consulting room.

'Put him on the table please,' I said, and as he lifted the little animal I decided that I couldn't let this opportunity pass. While I was carrying out my examination I would quite casually discuss recent events. Nothing nasty, no clever phrases, just a quiet probe into the situation. I was just about to say something like 'What's the idea of all those tricks you play on me?' when I took my first look at the dog and everything else fled from my mind.

He wasn't much more than a big puppy and an out-and-out mongrel. His shiny black coat could have come from a labrador and there was a suggestion of terrier in the pointed nose and pricked ears, but the long string-like tail and the knock-kneed fore limbs baffled me. For all that he was an attractive little creature with a sweetly expressive face.

But the things that seized my whole attention were the yellow blobs of pus in the corners of the eyes, the mucopurulent discharge from the nostrils and the photophobia which made the dog blink painfully at the light from the surgery window.

Classical canine distemper is so easy to diagnose but there is never any satisfaction in doing so.

'I didn't know you had a dog,' I said. 'How long have you had him?'

'A month. Feller got 'im from t'dog and cat home at Hartington and sold 'im to me.'

'I see.' I took the temperature and was not surprised to find it was 104 °F.

'How old is he?'

'Nine months.'

I nodded. Just about the worst age.

I went ahead and asked all the usual questions but I knew the answers already.

Yes, the dog had been slightly off colour for a week or two. No, he wasn't really ill, but listless and coughing occasionally. And of course it was not until the eyes and nose began to discharge that the boy became worried and brought him to see me. That was when we usually saw these cases – when it was too late.

Wesley imparted the information defensively, looking at me under lowered brows as though he expected me to clip his ear at any moment. But as I studied him any aggressive feelings I may have harboured evaporated quickly. The imp of hell appeared on closer examination to be a neglected child. His elbows stuck out through holes in a filthy jersey, his shorts were similarly ragged, but what appalled me most was the sour smell of his unwashed little body. I hadn't thought there were children like this in Darrowby.

When he had answered my questions he made an effort and blurted out one of his own.

'What's matter with 'im?'

I hesitated a moment. 'He's got distemper, Wes.'

'What's that?'

'Well, it's a nasty infectious disease. He must have got it from another sick dog.'

'Will 'e get better?'

'I hope so. I'll do the best I can for him.' I couldn't bring myself to tell a small boy of his age that his pet was probably going to die.

I filled a syringe with a 'mixed macterin' which we used at that time against the secondary invaders of distemper. It never did much good and even now with all our antibiotics we cannot greatly influence the final outcome. If you can catch a case in the early viral phase then a shot of hyperimmune serum is curative, but people rarely bring their dogs in until that phase is over.

As I gave the injection the dog whimpered a little and the boy stretched out a hand and patted him.

'It's awright, Duke,' he said.

'That's what you call him, is it – Duke?'

'Aye.' He fondled the ears and the dog turned, whipped his strange long tail about and licked the hand quickly. Wes smiled and looked up at me and for a moment the tough mask dropped from the grubby features and in the dark wild eyes I read sheer delight. I swore under my breath. This made it worse.

I tipped some boracic crystals into a box and handed it over. 'Use this dissolved in water to keep his eyes and nose clean. See how his nostrils are all caked and blocked up – you can make him a lot more comfortable.'

He took the box without speaking and almost with the same movement dropped three and sixpence on the table. It was about our average charge and resolved my doubts on that score.

'When'll ah bring 'im back?' he asked.

I looked at him doubtfully for a moment. All I could do was repeat the injections, but was it going to make the slightest difference?

The boy misread my hesitation.

'Ah can pay!' he burst out. 'Ah can get t'money!'

'Oh I didn't mean that, Wes. I was just wondering when it would be suitable. How about bringing him in on Thursday?'

He nodded eagerly and left with his dog.

As I swabbed the table with disinfectant I had the old feeling of helplessness. The modern veterinary surgeon does not see nearly as many cases of distemper as we used to, simply because most people immunize their puppies at the earliest possible moment. But back in the thirties it was only the fortunate dogs who were inoculated. The disease is so easy to prevent but almost impossible to cure.

The next three weeks saw an incredible change in Wesley Binks's character. He had built up a reputation as an idle scamp but now he was transformed into a model of industry, delivering papers in the mornings, digging people's gardens, helping to drive the beasts at the auction mart. I was perhaps the only one who knew he was doing it for Duke.

He brought the dog in every two or three days and paid on the nail. I naturally charged him as little as possible but the money he earned went on other things – fresh meat from the butcher, extra milk and biscuits.

'Duke's looking very smart today,' I said on one of the visits. 'I see you've been getting him a new collar and lead.'

The boy nodded shyly then looked up at me, dark eyes intent. 'Is 'e any better?'

'Well, he's about the same, Wes. That's how it goes – dragging on without much change.'

'When . . . when will ye know?'

I thought for a moment. Maybe he would worry less if he understood the situation. 'The thing is this. Duke will get better if he can avoid the nervous complications of distemper.'

'Wot's them?'

'Fits, paralysis and a thing called chorea which makes the muscles twitch.'

'Wot if he gets them?'

'It's a bad lookout in that case. But not all dogs develop them.' I tried to smile reassuringly. 'And there's one thing in Duke's favour – he's not a pure-bred. Cross-bred dogs have a thing called hybrid vigour which helps them to fight disease. After all, he's eating fairly well and he's quite lively, isn't he?'

'Aye, not bad.'

'Well then, we'll carry on. I'll give him another shot now.'

The boy was back in three days and I knew by his face he had momentous news.

'Duke's a lot better – 'is eyes and nose 'ave dried up and he's eatin' like a 'oss!' He was panting with excitement.

I lifted the dog on to the table. There was no doubt he was

enormously improved and I did my best to join in the rejoicing.

'That's great, Wes,' I said, but a warning bell was tinkling in my mind. If nervous symptoms were going to supervene, this was the time – just when the dog was apparently recovering.

I forced myself to be optimistic. 'Well now, there's no need to come back any more but watch him carefully and if you see anything unusual bring him in.'

The ragged little figure was overjoyed. He almost pranced along the passage with his pet and I hoped fervently that I would not see them in there again.

That was on the Friday evening and by Monday I had put the whole thing out of my head and into the category of satisfying memories when the boy came in with Duke on the lead.

I looked up from the desk where I was writing in the day book. 'What is it, Wes?'

'He's dotherin'.'

I didn't bother going through to the consulting room but hastened from behind the desk and crouched on the floor, studying the dog intently. At first I saw nothing, then as I watched I could just discern a faint nodding of the head. I placed my hand on the top of the skull and waited. And it was there; the slight but regular twitching of the temporal muscles which I had dreaded.

'I'm afraid he's got chorea, Wes.' I said.

'What's that?'

'It's one of the things I was telling you about. Sometimes they call it St Vitus' Dance. I was hoping it wouldn't happen.'

The boy looked suddenly small and forlorn and he stood there silent, twisting the new leather lead between his fingers. It was such an effort for him to speak that he almost closed his eyes.

'Will 'e die?'

'Some dogs do get over it, Wes. 'I didn't tell him that I had seen it happen only once. 'I've got some tablets which might help him. I'll get you some.'

56

I gave him a few of the arsenical tablets I had used in my only cure. I didn't even know if they had been responsible but I had nothing more to offer.

Duke's chorea pursued a text book course over the next two weeks. All the things which I had feared turned up in a relentless progression. The twitching spread from his head to his limbs, then his hindquarters began to sway as he walked.

His young master brought him in repeatedly and I went through the motions, trying at the same time to make it clear that it was all hopeless. The boy persisted doggedly, rushing about meanwhile with his paper deliveries and other jobs, insisting on paying though I didn't want his money. Then one afternoon he called in.

'Ah couldn't bring Duke,' he muttered. 'Can't walk now. Will you come and see 'im?'

We got into my car. It was a Sunday, about three o'clock and the streets were quiet. He led me up the cobbled yard and opened the door of one of the houses.

The stink of the place hit me as I went in. Country vets aren't easily sickened but I felt my stomach turning. Mrs Binks was very fat and a filthy dress hung shapelessly on her as she slumped, cigarette in mouth, over the kitchen table. She was absorbed in a magazine which lay in a clearing among mounds of dirty dishes and her curlers nodded as she looked up briefly at us.

On the couch under the window her husband sprawled asleep, open-mouthed, snoring out the reek of beer. The sink, which held a further supply of greasy dishes, was covered in a revolting green scum. Clothes, newspapers and nameless rubbish littered the floor and over everything a radio blasted away at full strength.

The only clean new thing was the dog basket in the corner. I went across and bent over the little animal. Duke was now prostrate and helpless, his body emaciated and jerking uncontrollably. The sunken eyes had filled up again with pus and gazed apathetically ahead.

'Wes,' I said. 'You've got to let me put him to sleep.'

He didn't answer, and as I tried to explain, the blaring radio drowned my words. I looked over at his mother.

'Do you mind turning the radio down?' I asked.

She jerked her head at the boy and he went over and turned the knob. In the ensuing silence I spoke to him again.

'It's the only thing, believe me. You can't let him die by inches like this.'

He didn't look at me. All his attention was fixed desperately on his dog. Then he raised a hand and I heard his whisper.

'Awright.'

I hurried out to the car for the Nembutal.

'I promise you he'll feel no pain,' I said as I filled the syringe. And indeed the little creature merely sighed before lying motionless, the fateful twitching stilled at last.

I put the syringe in my pocket. 'Do you want me to take him away, Wes?'

He looked at me bewilderedly and his mother broke in.

'Aye, get 'im out. Ah never wanted t'bloody thing 'ere in t'first place.' She resumed her reading.

I quickly lifted the little body and went out. Wes followed me and watched as I opened the boot and laid Duke gently on top of my black working coat.

As I closed the lid he screwed his knuckles into his eyes and his body shook. I put my arm across his shoulders, and as he leaned against me for a moment and sobbed I wondered if he had ever been able to cry like this – like a little boy with somebody to comfort him.

But soon he stood back and smeared the tears across the dirt on his cheeks.

'Are you going back into the house, Wes?' I asked.

He blinked and looked at me with a return of his tough expression.

'Naw!' he said and turned and walked away. He didn't look back and I watched him cross the road, climb a wall and trail away across the fields towards the river.

And it has always seemed to me that at that moment Wes walked back into his old life. From then on there were no more odd jobs or useful activities. He never played any more tricks on me but in other ways he progressed into more serious misdemeanours. He set barns on fire, was up before the magistrates for theft and by the time he was thirteen he was stealing cars.

Finally he was sent to an approved school and then he disappeared from the district. Nobody knew where he went and most people forgot him. One person who didn't was the police sergeant.

'That young Wesley Binks,' he said to me ruminatively. 'He was a wrong 'un if ever I saw one. You know, I don't think he ever cared a damn for anybody or any living thing in his life.'

'I know how you feel, sergeant,' I replied, 'But you're not entirely right. There was one living thing . . .'

six

Tristan would never have won any prizes as an exponent of the haute cuisine.

We got better food in the RAF than most people in wartime Britain but it didn't compare with the Darrowby fare. I suppose I had been spoiled; first by Mrs Hall, then by Helen. There were only brief occasions at Skeldale House when we did not eat like kings and one of those was when Tristan was installed as temporary cook.

It began one morning at breakfast in the days when I was still a bachelor and Tristan and I were taking our places at the mahogany dining table. Siegfried bustled in, muttered a greeting and began to pour his coffee. He was unusually distrait as he buttered a slice of toast and cut into one of the rashers on his plate, then after a minute's thoughtful chewing he brought down his hand on the table with a suddenness that made me jump.

'I've got it!' he exclaimed.

'Got what?' I enquired.

Siegfried put down his knife and fork and wagged a finger at me. 'Silly, really, I've been sitting here puzzling about what to do and it's suddenly clear.'

'Why, what's the trouble?'

'It's Mrs Hall,' he said. 'She's just told me her sister has been taken ill and she has to go and look after her. She thinks she'll be away for a week and I've been wondering who I could get to look after the house.'

'I see.'

'Then it struck me.' He sliced a corner from a fried egg. 'Tristan can do it.'

'Eh?' His brother looked up, startled, from his *Daily Mirror*. 'Me?'

'Yes, you! You spend a lot of time on your arse. A bit of useful activity would be good for you.'

Tristan looked at him warily. 'What do you mean – useful activity?'

'Well, keeping the place straight,' Siegfried said. 'I wouldn't expect perfection but you could tidy up each day, and of course prepare the meals.'

'Meals?'

'That's right.' Siegfried gave him a level stare. 'You can cook, can't you?'

'Well, er, yes . . . I can cook sausage and mash.'

Siegfried waved an expansive hand. 'There you are, you see, no problem. Push over those fried tomatoes, will you, James?'

I passed the dish silently. I had only half heard the conversation because part of my mind was far away. Just before breakfast I had had a phone call from Ken Billings, one of our best farmers, and his words were still echoing in my head.

'Mr Herriot, that calf you saw yesterday is dead. That's the third 'un I've lost in a week and I'm flummoxed. I want ye out here this mornin' to have another look round.'

I sipped my coffee absently. He wasn't the only one who was flummoxed. Three fine calves had shown symptoms of acute gastric pain, I had treated them and they had died.

That was bad enough but what made it worse was that I hadn't the faintest idea what was wrong with them.

I wiped my lips and got up quickly. 'Siegfried, I'd like to go to Billings' first. Then I've got the rest of the round you gave me.'

'Fine, James, by all means.' My boss gave me a sweet and encouraging smile, balanced a mushroom on a piece of fried bread and conveyed it to his mouth. He wasn't a big eater but he did love his breakfast.

On the way to the farm my mind beat about helplessly. What more could I do than I had already done? In these obscure cases one was driven to the conclusion that the animal had eaten something harmful. At times I had spent hours roaming around pastures looking for poisonous plants but that was pointless with Billings's calves because they had never been out; they were mere babies of a month old.

I had carried out post mortem examinations of the dead animals but had found only a non-specific gastro-enteritis. I had sent kidneys to the laboratory for lead estimation with negative result; like their owner, I was flummoxed.

Mr Billings was waiting for me in his yard.

'Good job I rang you!' he said breathlessly. 'There's another 'un startin'.'

I rushed with him into the buildings and found what I expected and dreaded; a small calf kicking at its stomach, getting up and down, occasionally rolling on its straw bed. Typical abdominal pain. But why?

I went over it as with the others. Temperature normal, lungs clear, only rumenal atony and extreme tenderness as I palpated the abdomen.

As I was putting the thermometer back in its case the calf suddenly toppled over and went into a frothing convulsion. Hastily I injected sedatives, calcium, magnesium, but with a feeling of doom. I had done it all before.

'What the hell is it?' the farmer asked, voicing my thoughts.

I shrugged. 'It's acute gastritis, Mr Billings, but I wish I knew the cause. I could swear this calf has eaten some irritant or corrosive poison.'

'Well, dang it, they've nobbut had milk and a few nuts.' The farmer spread his hands. 'There's nothing they can get to hurt them.'

Again, wearily, I went through the old routine; ferreting around in the calf pen, trying to find some clue. An old paint tin, a burst packet of sheep dip. It was amazing, the things you came across in the clutter of a farm building.

But not at Mr Billings's place. He was meticulously tidy, particularly with his calves, and the window sills and shelves were free from rubbish. It was the same with the milk buckets, scoured to spotless cleanliness after every feed.

Mr Billings had a thing about his calves. His two teenage sons were fanatically keen on farming and he encouraged them in all the agricultural skills; but he fed the calves himself.

'Feeding them calves is t'most important job in stock rearing,' he used to say. 'Get 'em over that first month and you're half way there.'

And he knew what he was talking about. His charges never suffered from the normal ailments of the young; no scour, no joint ill, no pneumonia. I had often marvelled at it, but it made the present disaster all the more unbearable.

'All right,' I said with false breeziness as I left. 'Maybe this one won't be so bad. Give me a ring in the morning.'

I did the rest of my round in a state of gloom and at lunch I was still so preoccupied that I wondered what had happened when Tristan served the meal. I had entirely forgotten about Mrs Hall's absence.

However, the sausage and mash wasn't at all bad and Tristan was lavish with his helpings. The three of us cleaned our plates pretty thoroughly, because morning is the busiest working time in practice and I was always famished by midday.

My mind was still on Mr Billings's problem during the afternoon calls and when we sat down to supper I was only mildly surprised to find another offering of sausage and mash.

'Same again, eh?' Siegfried grunted, but he got through his plateful and left without further comment.

The next day started badly. I came into the dining room to find the table bare and Siegfried stamping around.

'Where the hell is our breakfast?' he burst out. 'And where the hell is Tristan?'

He pounded along the passage and I heard his shouts in the kitchen 'Tristan! Tristan!'

I knew he was wasting his time. His brother often slept in and it was just a bit more noticeable this morning.

My boss returned along the passage at a furious gallop and I steeled myself for some unpleasantness as the young man was rousted from his bed. But Tristan, as usual, was master of the situation. Siegfried had just begun to take the stairs three at a time when his brother descended from the landing, knotting his tie with perfect composure. It was uncanny. He always got more than his share of sleeping time but was rarely caught between the sheets.

'Sorry, chaps,' he murmured. 'Afraid I overslept.'

'Yes, that's all right!' shouted Siegfried. 'But how about our bloody breakfast? I gave you a job to do!'

Tristan was contrite. 'I really do apologize, but I was up late last night, peeling potatoes.'

His brother's face flushed. 'I know all about that!' he barked. 'You didn't start till after closing time at the Drovers!'

'Well, that's right.' Tristan swallowed and his face assumed the familiar expression of pained dignity. 'I did feel a bit dry last night. Think it must have been all the cleaning and dusting I did.'

Siegfried did not reply. He shot a single exasperated look at the young man then turned to me. 'We'll have to make do with bread and marmalade this morning, James. Come through to the kitchen and we'll . . .'

The jangling telephone cut off his words. I lifted the receiver and listened and it must have been the expression on my face which stopped him in the doorway.

'What's the matter, James?' he asked as I came away from the phone. 'You look as though you've had a kick in the belly.'

I nodded. 'That's how I feel. That calf is nearly dead at

Billings's and there's another one ill. I wish you'd come out there with me, Siegfried.'

My boss stood very still as he looked over the side of the pen at the little animal. It didn't seem to know where to put itself, rising and lying down, kicking at some inward pain, writhing its hindquarters from side to side. As he watched it fell on its side and began to thrash around with all four limbs.

'James,' he said quietly. 'That calf has been poisoned.'

'That's what I thought, but how?'

Mr Billings broke in. 'It's no good talkin' like that, Mr Farnon. We've been over this place time and time again and there's nowt for them to get.'

'Well, we'll go over it again.' Siegfried stalked around the calf house as I had done and when he returned his face was expressionless.

'Where do you get the nuts from? he grunted, crumbling one of the cubes between his fingers.

Mr Billings threw his arms wide. 'From t'local mill. Ryders' best. You can't fault them, surely.'

Siegfried said nothing. Ryders were noted for their meticulous preparation of cattle food. He went over the sick calf with stethoscope and thermometer, digging his fingers into the hairy abdominal wall, staring impassively at the calf's face to note its reaction. He did the same with my patient of yesterday whose glazing eyes and cold extremities told their grim tale. Then he gave the calves almost the same treatment as I had and we left.

He was silent for the first half mile, then he beat the wheel suddenly with one hand. 'There's an irritant poison there, James! As sure as God made little apples there is. But I'm damned if I know where it's coming from.'

Our visit had taken a long time and we returned to Skeldale House for lunch. Like myself, his mind was still wrestling with Mr Billing's problem and he hardly winced as Tristan placed a steaming plateful of sausage and mash before him. Then, as he prodded the mash with a fork, he appeared to come to the surface.

'God almighty!' he exclaimed. 'Have we got this again?'

Tristan smiled ingratiatingly. 'Yes, indeed. Mr Johnson told me they were a particularly fine batch of sausages today. Definitely superior, he said.'

'Is that so?' His brother gave him a sour glance. 'Well, they look the bloody same to me. Like supper yesterday – and like lunch.' His voice began to rise, then he subsided.

'Oh, what the hell,' he muttered, and began to toy listlessly with the food. Clearly those calves had drained him and I knew how he felt.

I got through my share without much difficulty – I've always liked sausage and mash.

But my boss is a resilient character and when we met in the late afternoon he was bursting with his old spirit.

'That call to Billings's shook me, James, I can tell you.' he said. 'But I've revisited a few of my other cases since then and they're all improving nicely. Raises the morale tremendously. Here, let me get you a drink.'

He reached into the cupboard above the mantelpiece for the gin bottle and after pouring a couple of measures he looked benignly at his brother who was tidying the sitting room.

Tristan was making a big show, running a carpet sweeper up and down, straightening cushions, flicking a duster at everything in sight. He sighed and panted with effort as he bustled around, the very picture of a harassed domestic. He needed only a mob cap and frilly apron to complete the image.

We finished our drinks and Siegfried immersed himself in the *Veterinary Record* as savoury smells began to issue from the kitchen. It was about seven o'clock when Tristan put his head round the door.

'Supper is on the table,' he said.

My boss put down the *Record*, rose and stretched expansively. 'Good, I'm ready for it, too.'

I followed him into the dining room and almost cannoned into his back as he halted abruptly. He was staring in disbelief at the tureen in the middle of the table.

'Not bloody sausage and mash again!' he bellowed.

Tristan shuffled his feet. 'Well, er, yes – it's very nice really.'

'Very nice! I'm beginning to dream about the blasted stuff. Can't you cook anything else?'

'Well, I told you.' Tristan looked wounded. 'I told you I could cook sausage and mash.'

'Yes, you did!' shouted his brother. 'But you didn't say you couldn't cook anything else BUT sausage and bloody mash!'

Tristan made a non-committal gesture and his brother sank wearily down at the table.

'Go on, then,' he sighed. 'Dish it out and heaven help us.'

He took a small mouthful from his plate then gripped at his stomach and emitted a low moan. 'This stuff is killing me. I don't think I'll ever be the same after this week.'

The following day opened in dramatic fashion. I had just got out of bed and was reaching for my dressing gown when an explosion shook the house. It was a great 'WHUFF' which rushed like a mighty wind through passages and rooms, rattling the windows and leaving an ominous silence in its wake.

I dashed out to the landing and ran into Siegfried, who stared wide-eyed at me for a moment before galloping downstairs.

In the kitchen Tristan was lying on his back amid a litter of pans and dishes. Several rashers of bacon and a few smashed eggs nestled on the flags.

'What the hell's going on?' Siegfried shouted.

His brother looked up at him with mild interest. 'I really don't know. I was lighting the fire and there was a bang.'

'Lighting the fire . . .?'

'Yes, I've had a little difficulty these last two mornings. The thing wouldn't go. I think the chimney needs sweeping. These old houses . . .'

'Yes, yes!' Siegfried burst out. 'We know, but what the hell happened?'

Tristan sat up. Even then, among the debris with smuts all over his face, he still retained his poise. 'Well, I thought I'd hurry things along a bit,' (His agile mind was forever seeking new methods of conserving energy.) 'I soaked a piece of cotton wool in ether and chucked that in.'

'Ether?'

'Well yes, it's inflammable, isn't it?'

'Inflammable!' His brother was pop-eyed. 'It's bloody well explosive! It's a wonder you didn't blow the whole place up.'

Tristan rose and dusted himself off. 'Ah well, never mind. I'll soon have breakfast ready.'

'You can forget that.' Siegfried took a long shuddering breath then went over to the bread tin, extracted a loaf and began to saw at it. 'The breakfast's on the floor, and anyway, by the time you've cleared up this mess we'll be gone. Bread and marmalade all right for you, James?'

We went out together again. My boss had arranged that Ken Billings should postpone his calf feeding till we got there so that we could witness the process.

It wasn't a happy arrival. Both the calves had died and the farmer's eyes held a look of desperation.

Siegfried's jaw clenched tight for a moment then he motioned with his hand. 'Please carry on, Mr Billings. I want to see you feed them.'

The nuts were always available for the little animals but we watched intently as the farmer poured the milk into the buckets and the calves started to drink. The poor man had obviously given up hope and I could tell by his apathetic manner that he hadn't much faith in this latest ploy.

Neither had I, but Siegfried prowled up and down like a caged panther as though willing something to happen. The calves raised white-slobbered muzzles enquiringly as he hung over them but they could offer no more explanation of the mystery than I could myself.

I looked across the long row of pens. There were still more than thirty calves left in the building and the terrible thought arose that the disease might spread through all of them. My mind was recoiling when Siegfried stabbed a finger at one of the buckets.

'What's that?' he snapped.

The farmer and I went over and gazed down at a circular black object about half an inch across floating on the surface of the milk.

'Bit o' muck got in somehow,' Mr Billings mumbled. 'I'll 'ave it out.' He put his hand into the bucket.

'No, let me!' Siegfried carefully lifted the thing, shook the milk from his fingers and studied it with interest.

'This isn't muck,' he murmured. 'Look, it's concave – like a little cup.' He rubbed a corner between thumb and forefinger. 'I'll tell you what it is, it's a scab. Where the heck has it come from?'

He began to examine the neck and head of the calf, then became very still as he handled one of the little horn buds. 'There's a raw surface here. You can see where the scab belongs.' He placed the dark cup over the bud and it fitted perfectly.

The farmer shrugged. 'Aye, well, I can understand that. I disbudded all the calves about a fortnight sin'.'

'What did you use, Mr Billings?' My colleague's voice was soft.

'Oh, some new stuff. Feller came round sellin' it. You just paint it on – it's a lot easier than t'awd caustic stick.'

'Have you got the bottle?'

'Aye, it's in t'house. I'll get it.'

When the farmer returned Siegfried read the label and handed the bottle to me.

'Butter of antimony, Jim. Now we know.'

'But ... what are you on about?' asked the farmer bewilderedly.

Siegfried looked at him sympathetically. 'Antimony is a deadly poison, Mr Billings. Oh, it'll burn your horn buds off, all right, but if it gets in among the food, that's it.'

The farmer's eyes widened. 'Yes, dang it, and when they put their heads down to drink that's just when the scabs would fall off!'

'Exactly,' Siegfried said. 'Or they maybe knocked the horn buds on the sides of the bucket. Anyway, let's make sure the others are safe.'

We went round all the calves, removing the lethal crusts and scrubbing the buds clean, and when we finally drove away we knew that the brief but painful episode of the Billings calves was over.

In the car, my colleague put his elbow on the wheel and drove with his chin cupped in his hands. He often did this when in contemplative mood and it never failed to unnerve me.

'James,' he said, 'I've never seen anything like that before. It really is one for the book.'

His words were prophetic, for as I write about it now I realize that it has never been repeated in the thirty-five years that have passed since then.

At Skeldale House we parted to go our different ways. Tristan, no doubt anxious to redeem himself after the morning's explosive beginning, was plying mop and bucket and swabbing the passage with the zeal of one of Nelson's sailors.

But when Siegfried drove away, the activity stopped abruptly and as I was leaving with my pockets stuffed with the equipment for my round I glanced into the sitting room and saw the young man stretched in his favourite chair.

I went in and looked with some surprise at a pan of sausages balanced on the coals.

'What's this?' I asked.

Tristan lit a Woodbine, shook out his *Daily Mirror* and put his feet up. 'Just prepared lunch, old lad.'

'In here?'

'Yes, Jim, I've had enough of that hot stove – there's no comfort through there. And anyway, the kitchen's such a bloody long way away.'

I gazed down at the reclining form. 'No need to ask what's on the menu?'

'None at all, old son.' Tristan loked up from his paper with a seraphic smile.

I was about to leave when a thought struck me. 'Where are the potatoes?'

'In the fire.'

'In the fire!'

'Yes, I just popped them in there to roast for a while. They're delicious that way.'

'Are you sure?'

'Absolutely, Jim. I'll tell you – you'll fall in love with my cooking all over again.'

I didn't get back till nearly one o'clock. Tristan was not in the sitting room but a haze of smoke hung on the air and a reek like a garden bonfire prickled in my nostrils.

I found the young man in the kitchen. His *savoir faire* had vanished and he was prodding desperately at a pile of coal black spheres.

I stared at him. 'What are those?'

'The bloody potatoes, Jim! I fell asleep for a bit and this happened!'

He gingerly sawed through one of the objects. In the centre of the carbonaceous ball I could discern a small whitish marble which seemed to be all that remained of the original vegetable.

'Hell's bells, Triss! What are you going to do?'

He gave me a stricken glance. 'Hack out the centres and mash 'em up together. It's all I CAN do.'

This was something I couldn't bear to watch. I went upstairs, had a wash then took my place at the dining table. Siegfried was already seated and I could see that the little triumph of the morning had cheered him. He greeted me jovially.

'James, wasn't that the damndest thing at Ken Billings'? It's so satisfying to get it cleared up.'

But his smile froze as Tristan appeared and set down the tureens before him. From one peeped the inevitable sausages and the other contained an amorphous dark grey mass liberally speckled with black foreign bodies of varying size.

'What in the name of God,' he enquired with ominous quiet, 'is this?'

His brother swallowed. 'Sausage and mash,' he said lightly.

Siegfried gave him a cold look. 'I am referring to this.' He poked warily at the dark mound.

'Well, er, it's the potatoes.' Tristan cleared his throat. 'Got a little burnt, I'm afraid.'

My boss made no comment. With dangerous calm he spooned some of the material on to his plate, raised a forkful and began to chew slowly. Once or twice he winced as a particularly tough fragment of carbon cracked between his molars, then he closed his eyes and swallowed.

For a moment he was still, then he grasped his midriff with both hands, groaned and jumped to his feet.

'No, that's enough!' he cried. 'I don't mind investigating poisonings on the farms but I object to being poisoned myself in my own home!' He strode away from the table and paused at the door. 'I'm going over to the Drovers for lunch.'

As he left another spasm seized him. He clutched his stomach again and looked back.

'Now I know just how those poor bloody calves felt!'

seven

I suppose it was a little thoughtless of me to allow my scalpel to flash and flicker quite so close to Rory O'Hagan's fly buttons.

The incident came back to me as I sat in my room in St John's Wood reading Black's *Veterinary Dictionary*. It was a bulky volume to carry around and my RAF friends used to rib me about my 'vest pocket edition', but I had resolved to keep reading it in spare moments to remind me of my real life.

I had reached the letter 'C' and as the word 'Castration' looked up at me from the page I was jerked back to Rory.

I was castrating pigs. There were several litters to do and I was in a hurry and failed to notice the Irish farm worker's mounting apprehension. His young boss was catching the little animals and handing them to Rory who held them upside down, gripped between his thighs with their legs apart, and as I quickly incised the scrotums and drew out the testicles my blade almost touched the rough material of his trouser crutch.

'For God's sake, have a care, Mr Herriot!' he gasped at last.

I looked up from my work. 'What's wrong, Rory?'

'Watch what you're doin' with that bloody knife! You're whippin' it round between me legs like a bloody Red Indian. You'll do me a mischief afore you've finished!'

'Aye, be careful, Mr Herriot,' the young farmer cried. 'Don't geld Rory instead of the pig. His missus ud never forgive ye.' He burst into a loud peal of laughter, the Irishman grinned sheepishly and I giggled.

That was my undoing because the momentary inattention sent the blade slicing across my left forefinger. The razor-sharp edge went deep and in an instant the entire neighbourhood seemed flooded with my blood. I thought I would never staunch the flow. The red ooze continued, despite a long session of self-doctoring from the car boot, and when I finally drove away my finger was swathed in the biggest, clumsiest dressing I had ever seen. I had finally been forced to apply a large pad of cotton wool held in place with an enormous length of three-inch bandage.

It was dark when I left the farm: about five o'clock on a late December day, the light gone early and the stars beginning to show in a frosty sky. I drove slowly, the enormous finger jutting upwards from the wheel, pointing the way between the headlights like a guiding beacon. I was within half a mile of Darrowby with the lights of the little town beginning to wink between the bare roadside branches when a car approached, went past, then I heard a squeal of brakes as it stopped and began to double back.

It passed me again, drew into the side and I saw a frantically waving arm. I pulled up and a young man jumped from the driving seat and ran towards me.

He pushed his head in at the window. 'Are you the vet?' His voice was breathless, panic-stricken.

'Yes, I am.'

'Oh thank God! We're passing through on the way to Manchester and we've been to your surgery . . . they said you were out this way . . . described your car. Please help us!'

'What's the trouble?'

'It's our dog . . . in the back of the car. He's got a ball stuck in his throat. I . . . I think he might be dead.'

I was out of my seat and running along the road before he had finished. It was a big white saloon and in the darkness of the back seat a wailing chorus issued from several little heads silhoutted against the glass.

I tore open the door and the wailing took on words.

'Oh Benny, Benny, Benny . . .!'

I dimly discerned a large dog spread over the knees of four small children. 'Oh Daddy, he's dead, he's dead!'

'Let's have him out,' I gasped, and as the young man pulled on the forelegs I supported the body, which slid and toppled on to the tarmac with a horrible limpness.

I pawed at the hairy form. 'I can't see a bloody thing! Help me pull him round.'

We dragged the unresisting bulk into the headlights' glare and I could see it all. A huge, beautiful collie in his luxuriant prime, mouth gaping, tongue lolling, eyes staring lifelessly at nothing. He wasn't breathing.

The young father took one look then gripped his head with both hands. 'Oh God, oh God. . . .' From within the car I heard the quiet sobbing of his wife and the piercing cries from the back. 'Benny . . . Benny. . . .'

I grabbed the man's shoulder and shouted at him. 'What did you say about a ball?'

'It's in his throat . . . I've had my fingers in his mouth for ages but I couldn't move it.' The words came mumbling up from beneath the bent head.

I pushed my hand into the mouth and I could feel it all right. A sphere of hard solid rubber not much bigger than a golf ball and jammed like a cork in the pharynx, effectively

73

blocking the trachea. I scrabbled feverishly at the wet smoothness but there was nothing to get hold of. It took me about three seconds to realize that no human agency would ever get the ball out that way and without thinking I withdrew my hands, braced both thumbs behind the angle of the lower jaw and pushed.

The ball shot forth, bounced on the frosty road and rolled sadly on to the grass verge. I touched the corneal surface of the eye. No reflex. I slumped to my knees, burdened by the hopeless regret that I hadn't had the chance to do this just a bit sooner. The only function I could perform now was to take the body back to Skeldale House for disposal. I couldn't allow the family to drive to Manchester with a dead dog. But I wished fervently that I had been able to do more, and as I passed my hand along the richly coloured coat over the ribs the vast bandaged finger stood out like a symbol of my helplessness.

It was when I was gazing dully at the finger, the heel of my hand resting in an intercostal space, that I felt the faintest flutter from below.

I jerked upright with a hoarse cry. 'His heart's still beating! He's not gone yet!' I began to work on the dog with all I had. And out there in the darkness of that lonely country road it wasn't much. No stimulant injections, no oxygen cylinders or intratracheal tubes. But I depressed his chest with my palms every three seconds in the old-fashioned way, willing the dog to breathe as the eyes still stared at nothing. Every now and then I blew desperately down the throat or probed between the ribs for that almost imperceptible beat.

I don't know which I noticed first, the slight twitch of an eyelid or the small lift of the ribs which pulled the icy Yorkshire air into his lungs. Maybe they both happened at once but from that moment everything was dreamlike and wonderful. I lost count of time as I sat there while the breathing became deep and regular and the animal began to be aware of his surroundings; and by the time he started to look around him and twitch his tail tentatively I realized suddenly that I was stiff-jointed and almost frozen to the spot.

With some difficulty I got up and watched in disbelief as the collie staggered to his feet. The young father ushered him round to the back where he was received with screams of delight.

The man seemed stunned. Throughout the recovery he had kept muttering, 'You just flicked that ball out . . . just flicked it out. Why didn't I think of that . . . ?' And when he turned to me before leaving he appeared to be still in a state of shock.

'I don't . . . I don't know how to thank you,' he said huskily. 'It's a miracle.' He leaned against the car for a second. 'And now what is your fee? How much do I owe you?'

I rubbed my chin. I had used no drugs. The only expenditure had been time.

'Five bob,' I said. 'And never let him play with such a little ball again.'

He handed the money over, shook my hand and drove away. His wife, who had never left her place, waved as she left, but my greatest reward was in the last shadowy glimpse of the back seat where little arms twined around the dog, hugging him ecstatically, and in the cries, thankful and joyous, fading into the night.

'Benny . . . Benny . . . Benny. . . .'

Vets often wonder after a patient's recovery just how much credit they might take. Maybe it would have got better without treatment – it happened sometimes; it was difficult to be sure.

But when you know without a shadow of a doubt that, even without doing anything clever, you have pulled an animal back from the brink of death into the living, breathing world, it is a satisfaction which lingers, flowing like balm over the discomforts and frustrations of veterinary practice, making everything right.

Yet, in the case of Benny the whole thing had an unreal quality. I never even glimpsed the faces of those happy children nor that of their mother huddled in the front seat. I had a vague impression of their father but he had spent most of the time with his head in his hands. I wouldn't have known him if I met him in the street. Even the dog, in the unnatural glare of the headlights, was a blurred memory.

It seemed the family had the same feeling because a week later I had a pleasant letter from the mother. She apologized for skulking out of the way so shamelessly, she thanked me for saving the life of their beloved dog who was now prancing around with the children as though nothing had happened, and she finished with the regret that she hadn't even asked me my name.

Yes, it had been a strange episode, and not only were those people unaware of my name but I'd like to bet they would fail to recognize me if they saw me again.

In fact, looking back at the affair, the only thing which stood out unequivocal and substantial was my great white-bound digit which had hovered constantly over the scene, almost taking on a personality and significance of its own. I am sure that is what the family remembered best about me because of the way the mother's letter began.

'Dear Vet with the bandaged finger . . .'

eight

My stint in London was nearing its end. Our breaking-in weeks were nearly over and we waited for news of posting to Initial Training Wing.

The air was thick with rumours. We were going to Aberystwyth in Wales; too far away for me, I wanted the north. Then we were going to Newquay in Cornwall; worse still. I was aware that the impending birth of AC2 Herriot's child did not influence the general war strategy but I still wanted to be as near to Helen as possible at the time.

The whole London phase is blurred in my memory. Possibly because everything was so new and different that the impressions could not be fully absorbed, and also perhaps because I was tired most of the time. I think we were all tired. Few of us were used to being jerked from slumber at 6 a.m. every morning and spending the day in continual physical activity. If we weren't being drilled we were being marched to meals, to classes, to talks. I had lived in a motor car for a few years and the rediscovery of my legs was painful.

There were times, too, when I wondered what it was all about. Like all the other young men I had imagined that after a few brisk preliminaries I would be sitting in an aeroplane, learning to fly, but it turned out that this was so far in the future that it was hardly mentioned. At the ITW we would spend months learning navigation, principles of flight, morse and many other things.

I was thankful for one blessing. I had passed the mathematics exam. I have always counted on my fingers and still do and I had been so nervous about this that I went to classes with the ATC in Darrowby before my call-up, dredging from my schooldays horrific calculations about trains passing each other at different speeds and water running in and out of bath tubs. But I had managed to scrape through and felt ready to face anything.

There were some unexpected shocks in London. I didn't anticipate spending days mucking out some of the dirtiest piggeries I had ever seen. Somebody must have had the idea of converting all the RAF waste food into pork and bacon and of course there was plenty of labour at hand. I had a strong feeling of unreality as, with other aspiring pilots, I threw muck and swill around hour after hour.

There was another time I had the same feeling. One night three of us decided to go to the cinema. We took pains to get to the front of the queue for the evening meal so that we would be in time for the start of the picture. When the doors of the huge dining room at the zoo were thrown open we were first in, but a sergeant cook met us in the entrance with:

'I want three volunteers for dishwashing – you, you and you,' and marched us away.

He probably had a kind heart because he patted our shoulders as we climbed miserably into greasy dungarees.

'Never mind, lads,' he said. 'I'll see you get a real good meal afterwards.'

My friends were taken somewhere else and I found myself alone in a kind of dungeon at the end of a metal chute. Very soon dirty plates began to cascade down the chute and my job was to knock the food remains off them and transfer them to a mechanical washer.

The menu that night was cottage pie and chips, a combination which has remained engraved on my memory. For more than two hours I stood at bay while a nonstop torrent of crockery poured down on me; thousands and thousands of plates, every one bearing a smear of cottage pie, a blob of cold gravy, a few adhering chips.

As I reeled around in the meaty steam a little tune tinkled repetitively in my mind; it was the song Siegfried and I were forever singing as we waited to enter the RAF, the popular jingle which in our innocence we thought typified the new life ahead.

If I only had wings,
Oh what a difference it would make to things,
All day long I'd be in the sky, up on high,
Talking to the birdies that pass me by.

But in this reeking cavern with my hands, face, hair and every pore of my skin impregnated with cottage pie and chips, those birdies seemed far away.

At last, however, the plates began to slow down and finally stopped coming. The sergeant came in beaming and congratulated me on doing a fine job. He led me back to the dining hall, vast and empty save for my two friends. They both wore bemused, slightly stunned expressions and I am pretty sure I looked the same.

'Sit down here, lads,' the sergeant said. We took our places side by side in a corner with the bare boards of the table stretching away into the distance. 'I told you you'd get a real good meal, didn't I? Well, here it is.' He slid three heaped platefuls in front of us.

'There y'are,' he said. 'Cottage pie and chips, double helpin's!'

The following day I might have felt more disenchanted than ever, but news of the posting blotted out all other feelings. It seemed too good to be true – I was going to Scarborough. I had been there and I knew it as a beautiful seaside resort, but that wasn't why I was so delighted. It was because it was in Yorkshire.

nine

As we marched out of the station into the streets of Scarborough I could hardly believe I was back in Yorkshire. But if there had been any doubt in my mind it would have been immediately resolved by my first breath of the crisp, tangy air. Even in winter there had been no 'feel' to the soft London air and I half closed my eyes as I followed the tingle all the way down to my lungs.

Mind you, it was cold. Yorkshire is a cold place and I could remember the sensation almost of shock at the start of my first winter in Darrowby.

It was after the first snow and I followed the clanging ploughs up the Dale, bumping along between high white mounds till I reached old Mr Stokill's gate. With my fingers on the handle I looked through the glass at the new world beneath me. The white blanket rolled down the hillside and lapped over the roofs of the dwelling and outbuildings of the little farm. Beyond, it smoothed out and concealed the familiar features, the stone walls bordering the fields, the stream on the valley floor, turning the whole scene into something unknown and exciting.

But the thrill I felt at the strange beauty was swept away as I got out and the wind struck me. It was an Arctic blast screaming from the east, picking up extra degrees of cold as it drove over the frozen white surface. I was wearing a heavy overcoat and woollen gloves but the gust whipped its way right into my bones. I gasped and leaned my back against the car while I buttoned the coat up under my chin, then I struggled forward to where the gate shook and rattled. I fought it open and my feet crunched as I went through.

Coming round the corner of the byre I found Mr Stokill forking muck on to a heap, making a churned brown trail across the whiteness.

'Now then,' he muttered along the side of a half-smoked cigarette. He was over seventy but still ran the smallholding single-handed. He told me once that he had worked as a farm hand for six shillings a day for thirty years, yet still managed to save enough to buy his own little place. Maybe that was why he didn't want to share it.

'How are you, Mr Stokill?' I said, but just then the wind tore through the yard, clutching icily at my face, snatching my breath away so that I turned involuntarily to one side with an explosive 'Aaahh!'

The old farmer looked at me in surprise, then glanced around as though he had just noticed the weather.

'Aye, blows a bit thin this mornin', lad.' Sparks flew from the end of his cigarette as he leaned for a moment on the fork.

He didn't seem to have much protection against the cold. A light khaki smock fluttered over a ragged navy waistcoat, clearly once part of his best suit, and his shirt bore neither collar nor stud. The white stubble on his fleshless jaw was a reproach to my twenty-four years and suddenly I felt an inadequate city-bred softie.

The old man dug his fork into the manure pile and turned towards the buildings. 'Ah've got a nice few cases for ye to see today. Fust 'un's in 'ere.' He opened a door and I staggered gratefully into a sweet bovine warmth where a few shaggy little bullocks stood hock deep in straw.

'That's the youth we want.' He pointed to a dark roan

standing with one hind foot knuckled over. 'He's been on three legs for a couple o' days. Ah reckon he's got foul.'

I walked up to the little animal but he took off at a speed which made light of his infirmity.

'We'll have to run him into the passage. Mr Stokill,' I said. 'Just open the gate, will you?'

With the rough timbers pushed wide I got behind the bullock and sent him on to the opening. It seemed as though he was going straight through but at the entrance he stopped peeped into the passage and broke away. I galloped a few times round the yard after him, then had another go. The result was the same. After half a dozen tries I wasn't cold any more. I'll back chasing young cattle against anything else for working up a sweat, and I had already forgotten the uncharitable world outside. And I could see I was going to get warmer still because the bullock was beginning to enjoy the game, kicking up his heels and frisking around after each attempt.

I put my hands on my hips, waited till I got my breath back then turned to the farmer.

'This is hopeless. He'll never go in there,' I said. 'We'd maybe better try to get a rope on him.'

'Nay, lad, there's no need for that. We'll get him through t'gate right enough.' The old man ambled to one end of the yard and returned with an armful of clean straw. He sprinkled it freely in the gate opening and beyond in the passage, then turned to me. 'Now send 'im on.'

I poked a finger into the animal's rump and he trotted forward, proceeded unhesitatingly between the posts and into the passage.

Mr Stokill must have noticed my look of bewilderment.

'Aye, 'e just didn't like t'look of them cobbles. Once they was covered over he was awright.'

'Yes ... yes ... I see.' I followed the bullock slowly through.

He was indeed suffering from foul of the foot, the mediaeval term given because of the stink of the necrotic tissue between the cleats, and I didn't have any antibiotics or sulphonamides to treat it. It is so nice and easy these days to give an injection, knowing that the beast will be sound in a day or two. But all I could do was wrestle with the lunging hind foot, dressing the infected cleft with a crude mixture of copper sulphate and Stockholm tar and finishing with a pad of cotton wool held by a tight bandage. When I had finished I took off my coat and hung it on a nail. I didn't need it any more.

Mr Stokill looked approvingly at the finished job. 'Capital, capital,' he murmured. 'Now there's some little pigs in this pen got a bit o' scour. I want you to give 'em a jab wi' your needle.'

We had various *E coli* vaccines which sometimes did a bit of good in these cases and I entered the pen hopefully. But I left in a hurry because the piglets' mother didn't approve of a stranger wandering among her brood and she came at me open-mouthed, barking explosively. She looked as big as a donkey and when the cavernous jaws with the great yellowed teeth brushed my thigh I knew it was time to go. I hopped rapidly into the yard and crashed the door behind me.

I peered back ruminatively into the pen. 'We'll have to get her out of there before I can do anything, Mr Stokill.'

'Aye, you're right, young man, ah'll shift 'er.' He began to shuffle away.

I held up a hand. 'No, it's all right, I'll do it.' I couldn't let this frail old man go in there and maybe get knocked down and savaged, and I looked around for a means of protection. There was a battered shovel standing against a wall and I seized it.

'Open the door, please,' I said. 'I'll soon have her out.'

Once more inside the pen I held the shovel in front of me and tried to usher the huge sow towards the door. But my efforts at poking her rear end were fruitless; she faced me all the time, wide-mouthed and growling as I circled. When she got the blade of the shove between her teeth and began to worry it I called a halt.

As I left the pen I saw Mr Stokill dragging a large object over the cobbles.

'What's that?' I asked.

'Dustbin,' the old man grunted in reply.

'Dustbin! What on earth . . . ?'

He gave no further explanation but entered the pen. As the sow came at him he allowed her to run her head into the bin then, bent double, he began to back her towards the open door. The animal was clearly baffled. Suddenly finding herself in this strange dark place she naturally tried to retreat from it and all the farmer did was guide her.

Before she knew what was happening she was out in the yard. The old man calmly removed the bin and beckoned to me. 'Right you are, Mr Herriot, you can get on now.'

It had taken about twenty seconds.

Well, that was a relief, and anyway I knew what to do next. Lifting a sheet of corrugated iron which the farmer had ready I rushed in among the little pigs. I would pen them in a corner and the job would be over in no time.

But their mother's irritation had been communicated to the family. It was a big litter and there were sixteen of them hurtling around like little pink racehorses. I spent a long time diving frantically after them, jamming the sheet at a bunch only to see half of them streaking out the other end, and I might have gone on indefinitely had I not felt a gentle touch on my arm.

'Haud on, young man, haud on.' The old farmer looked at me kindly. 'If you'll nobbut stop runnin' after 'em they'll settle down. Just bide a minute.'

Slightly breathless, I stood by his side and listened as he addressed the little creatures.

'Giss-giss, giss-giss,' murmured Mr Stokill without moving. 'Giss-giss, giss-giss.'

The piglets slowed their headlong gallop to a trot, then, as though controlled by telepathy, they all stopped at once and stood in a pink group in one corner.

'Giss-giss,' said Mr Stokill approvingly, advancing almost imperceptibly with the sheet. 'Giss-giss.'

He unhurriedly placed the length of metal across the corner and jammed his foot against the bottom.

'Now then, put the toe of your wellington against t'other end and we 'ave 'em,' he said quietly.

After that the injection of the litter was a matter of a few minutes. Mr Stokill didn't say, 'Well, I'm teaching you a thing or two today, am I not?' There was no hint of triumph or self-congratulation in the calm old eyes. All he said was, 'I'm keepin' you busy this mornin', young man. I want you to look at a cow now. She's got a pea in her tit.'

'Peas' and other obstructions in the teats were very common in the days of hand milking. Some of them were floating milk calculi, others tiny pedunculated tumours, injuries to the teat lining, all sorts of things. It was a whole diverting little field in itself and I approached the cow with interest.

But I didn't get very near before Mr Stokill put his hand on my shoulder.

'Just a minute, Mr Herriot, don't touch 'er tit yet or she'll clout ye. She's an awd bitch. Wait a minute till ah rope 'er.'

'Oh right,' I said. 'But I'll do it.'

He hesitated. 'Ah reckon I ought to . . .'

'No, no, Mr Stokill that's quite unnecessary, I know how to stop a cow kicking.' I said primly. 'Kindly hand me that rope.'

'But . . . she's a bugger . . . kicks like a 'oss. She's a right good milker but . . .'

'Don't worry,' I said, smiling. 'I'll stop her little games.'

I began to unwind the rope. It was good to be able to demonstrate that I did know something about handling animals even though I had been qualified for only a few months. And it made a change to be told before and not after the job that a cow was a kicker. A cow once kicked me nearly to the other end of the byre and as I picked myself up the farmer said unemotionally, 'Aye, she's allus had a habit o' that.'

Yes, it was nice to be warned, and I passed the rope round the animal's body in front of the udder and pulled it tight in a slip knot. Just like they taught us at college. She was a scrawny red shorthorn with a woolly poll and she regarded me with a contemplative eye as I bent down.

'All right, lass,' I said soothingly, reaching under her and gently grasping the teat. I squirted a few jets of milk then something blocked the end. Ah yes, there it was, quite large and unattached. I felt sure I could work it through the orifice without cutting the sphincter.

I took a firmer grip, squeezed tightly and immediately a cloven foot shot out like a whip lash and smacked me solidly on the knee. It is a particularly painful spot to be kicked and I spent some time hopping round the byre and cursing in a fervent whisper.

The farmer followed me anxiously. 'Ee, ah'm sorry, Mr Herriot, she's a right awd bugger. Better let me . . .'

I held up a hand. 'No, Mr Stokill. I already have her roped. I just didn't tie it tight enough, that's all.' I hobbled back to the animal, loosened the knot then retied it, pulling till my eyes popped. When I had finished, her abdomen was lifted high and nipped in like a wasp-waisted Victorian lady of fashion.

'That'll fix you,' I grunted, and bent to my work again. A few spurts of milk then the thing was at the teat end again, a pinkish-white object peeping through the orifice. A little extra pressure and I would be able to fish it out with the hypodermic needle I had poised ready. I took a breath and gripped hard.

This time the hoof caught me half way up the shin bone. She hadn't been able to get so much height into it but it was just as painful. I sat down on a milking stool, rolled up my trouser leg and examined the roll of skin which hung like a diploma at the end of a long graze where the sharp hoof had dragged along.

'Now then, you've 'ad enough, young man.' Mr Stokill removed my rope and gazed at me with commiseration. 'Ordinary methods don't work with this 'un. I 'ave to milk her twice a day and ah knaw.'

He fetched a soiled length of plough cord which had obviously seen much service and fastened it round the cow's hock. The other end had a hook which he fitted into a ring on the byre wall. It was just the right length to stretch taut, pulling the leg slightly back.

The old man nodded. 'Now try.'

With a feeling of fatalism I grasped the teat again. And it was as if the cow knew she was beaten. She never moved as I nipped hard and winkled out the offending obstruction. She couldn't do a thing about it.

'Ah, thank ye, lad,' the farmer said. 'That's champion. Been bothering me a bit has that. Didn't know what it was.' He held up a finger. 'One last job for ye. A young heifer with a bit o' stomach trouble, ah think. Saw her last night and she was a bit blown. She's in an outside buildin'.'

I put on my coat and we went out to where the wind welcomed us with savage glee. As the knife-like blast hit me, whistling up my nose and making my eyes water, I cowered in the lee of the stable.

'Where is this heifer?' I gasped.

Mr Stokill did not reply immediately. He was lighting another cigarette, apparently oblivious of the elements. He clamped the lid on an ancient brass lighter and jerked his thumb.

'Across the road. Up there.'

I followed his gesture over the buried walls, across the narrow roadway between the ploughed-out snow dunes to where the fell rose steeply in a sweep of broken white to join the leaden sky. Unbroken, that is, except for a tiny barn, a grey stone speck just visible on the last airy swell hundreds of feet up where the hillside joined the moorland above.

'Sorry,' I said, still crouching against the wall. 'I can't see anything.'

The old man, lounging in the teeth of the wind, looked at me in surprise. 'You can't? Why, t'barn's good enough to see, isn't it?'

'The barn?' I pointed a shaking finger at the heights. 'You mean that building? The heifer's surely not in there!'

'Aye, she is. Ah keep a lot o' me young beasts in them spots.'

'But . . . but . . .' I was gabbling now. 'We'll never get up there! That snow's three feet deep!'

He blew smoke pleasurably from his nostrils. 'We will, don't tha worry. Just hang on a second.'

He disappeared into the stable and after a few moments I peeped inside. He was saddling a fat brown cob and I stared as he led the little animal out, climbed stiffly on to a box and mounted.

Looking down at me he waved cheerfully. 'Well, let's be goin'. Have you got your stuff?'

Bewilderedly I filled my pockets. A bottle of bloat mixture, a trochar and cannula, a packet of gentian and nux vomica. I did it in the dull knowledge that there was no way I could get up that hill.

On the other side of the road an opening had been dug and Mr Stokill rode through. I slithered in his wake, looking up hopelessly at the great smooth wilderness rearing above us.

Mr Stokill turned in the saddle. 'Get haud on t'tail,' he said.

'I beg your pardon?'

'Get a haud of 'is tail.'

As in a dream I seized the bristly hairs.

'No, both 'ands,' the farmer said patiently.

'That's grand, lad. Now 'ang on.'

He clicked his tongue, the cob plodded resolutely forward and so did I.

And it was easy! The whole world fell away beneath us as we soared upwards, and leaning back and enjoying it I watched the little valley unfold along its twisting length until I could see away into the main Dale with the great hills billowing round and white into the dark clouds.

At the barn the farmer dismounted. 'All right, young man?'

'All right, Mr Stokill.' As I followed him into the little building I smiled to myself. This old man had once told me that he left school when he was twelve, whereas I had spent most of the twenty-four years of my life in study. Yet when I looked back on the last hour or so I could come to only one conclusion.

He knew a lot more than I did.

ten

I had plenty of company for Christmas that year. We were billeted in the Grand Hotel, the massive Victorian pile which dominated Scarborough in turreted splendour from its eminence above the sea, and the big dining room was packed with several hundred shouting airmen. The iron discipline was relaxed for a few hours to let the Yuletide spirit run free.

It was so different from other Christmases I had known that it ought to have remained like a beacon in my mind, but I know that my strongest memory of Christmas will always be bound up with a certain little cat.

I first saw her when I was called to see one of Mrs Ainsworth's dogs, and I looked in some surprise at the furry black creature sitting before the fire.

'I didn't know you had a cat,' I said.

The lady smiled. 'We haven't, this is Debbie.'

'Debbie?'

'Yes, at least that's what we call her. She's a stray. Comes here two or three times a week and we give her some food. I don't know where she lives but I believe she spends a lot of her time around one of the farms along the road.'

'Do you ever get the feeling that she wants to stay with you?'

'No.' Mrs Ainsworth shook her head. 'She's a timid little thing. Just creeps in, has some food then flits away. There's something so appealing about her but she doesn't seem to want to let me or anybody into her life.'

I looked again at the little cat. 'But she isn't just having food today.'

'That's right. It's a funny thing but every now and again she slips through here into the lounge and sits by the fire for a few minutes. It's as though she was giving herself a treat.'

'Yes . . . I see what you mean.' There was no doubt there was something unusual in the attitude of the little animal. She was sitting bolt upright on the thick rug which lay before the fireplace in which the coals glowed and flamed. She made no effort to curl up or wash herself or do anything other than gaze quietly ahead. And there was something in the dusty black of her coat, the half-wild scrawny look of her, that gave me a clue. This was a special event in her life, a rare and wonderful thing; she was lapping up a comfort undreamed of in her daily existence.

As I watched she turned, crept soundlessly from the room and was gone.

'That's always the way with Debbie,' Mrs Ainsworth laughed. 'She never stays more than ten minutes or so, then she's off.'

She was a plumpish, pleasant-faced woman in her forties and the kind of client veterinary surgeons dream of; well off, generous, and the owner of three cosseted basset hounds. And it only needed the habitually mournful expressions of one of the dogs to deepen a little and I was round there post haste. Today one of the bassets had raised its paw and scratched its ear a couple of times and that was enough to send its mistress scurrying to the phone in great alarm.

So my visits to the Ainsworth home were frequent but undemanding, and I had ample opportunity to look out for the little cat which had intrigued me. On one occasion I spotted her nibbling daintily from a saucer at the kitchen door. As I watched she turned and almost floated on light footsteps into the hall then through the lounge door.

The three bassets were already in residence, draped snoring on the fireside rug, but they seemed to be used to Debbie because two of them sniffed her in a bored manner and the third merely cocked a sleepy eye at her before flopping back on the rich pile.

Debbie sat among them in her usual posture; upright, intent, gazing absorbedly into the glowing coals. This time I tried to make friends with her. I approached her carefully but she leaned away as I stretched out my hand. However, by patient wheedling and soft talk I managed to touch her and gently stroked her cheek with one finger. There was a moment when she responded by putting her head on one side and rubbing back against my hand but soon she was ready to leave. Once outside the house she darted quickly along the road then through a gap in a hedge and the last I saw was the little black figure flitting over the rain-swept grass of a field.

'I wonder where she goes,' I murmured half to myself.

Mrs Ainsworth appeared at my elbow. 'That's something we've never been able to find out.'

It must have been nearly three months before I heard from Mrs Ainsworth, and in fact I had begun to wonder at the bassets' long symptomless run when she came on the phone.

It was Christmas morning and she was apologetic. 'Mr Herriot, I'm so sorry to bother you today of all days. I should think you want a rest at Christmas like anybody else.' But her natural politeness could not hide the distress in her voice.

'Please don't worry about that,' I said. 'Which one is it this time?'

'It's not one of the dogs. It's . . . Debbie.'

'Debbie? She's at your house now?'

'Yes . . . but there's something wrong. Please come quickly.'

Driving through the market place I thought again that Darrowby on Christmas Day was like Dickens come to life; the empty square with the snow thick on the cobbles and hanging from the eaves of the fretted lines of roofs; the shops closed and the coloured lights of the Christmas trees winking at the windows of the clustering houses, warmly inviting against the cold white bulk of the fells behind.

Mrs Ainsworth's home was lavishly decorated with tinsel and holly, rows of drinks stood on the sideboard and the rich aroma of turkey and sage and onion stuffing wafted from the kitchen. But her eyes were full of pain as she led me through to the lounge.

Debbie was there all right, but this time everything was different. She wasn't sitting upright in her usual position; she was stretched quite motionless on her side, and huddled close to her lay a tiny black kitten.

I looked down in bewilderment. 'What's happened here?'

'It's the strangest thing,' Mrs Ainsworth replied. 'I haven't seen her for several weeks then she came in about two hours ago – sort of staggered into the kitchen, and she was carrying the kitten in her mouth. She took it through to the lounge and laid it on the rug and at first I was amused. But I could see all was not well because she sat as she usually does, but for a long time – over half an hour – then she lay down like this and she hasn't moved.'

I knelt on the rug and passed my hand over Debbie's neck and ribs. She was thinner than ever, her fur dirty and mud-caked. She did not resist as I gently opened her mouth. The tongue and mucous membranes were abnormally pale and the lips ice-cold against my fingers. When I pulled down her eyelid and saw the dead white conjunctiva a knell sounded in my mind.

I palpated the abdomen with a grim certainty as to what I would find and there was no surprise, only a dull sadness as my fingers closed around a hard lobulated mass deep among the viscera. Massive lymphosarcoma. Terminal and hopeless. I put my stethoscope on her heart and listened to the increasingly faint, rapid beat then I straightened up and sat on the rug looking sightlessly into the fireplace, feeling the warmth of the flames on my face.

Mrs Ainsworth's voice seemed to come from afar. 'Is she ill, Mr Herriot?'

I hesitated. 'Yes . . . yes, I'm afraid so. She has a malignant growth.' I stood up. 'There's absolutely nothing I can do. I'm sorry.'

'Oh!' Her hand went to her mouth and she looked at me wide-eyed. When at last she spoke her voice trembled. 'Well, you must put her to sleep immediately. It's the only thing to do. We can't let her suffer.'

'Mrs Ainsworth,' I said. 'There's no need. She's dying now – in a coma – far beyond suffering.'

She turned quickly away from me and was very still as she fought with her emotions. Then she gave up the struggle and dropped on her knees beside Debbie.

'Oh, poor little thing!' she sobbed and stroked the cat's

head again and again as the tears fell unchecked on the matted fur. 'What she must have come through. I feel I ought to have done more for her.'

For a few moments I was silent, feeling her sorrow, so discordant among the bright seasonal colours of this festive room. Then I spoke gently.

'Nobody could have done more than you,' I said. 'Nobody could have been kinder.'

'But I'd have kept her here – in comfort. It must have been terrible out there in the cold when she was so desperately ill – I daren't think about it. And having kittens, too – I . . . I wonder how many she did have?'

I shrugged. 'I don't suppose we'll ever know. Maybe just this one. It happens sometimes. And she brought it to you, didn't she?'

'Yes . . . that's right . . . she did . . . she did.' Mrs Ainsworth reached out and lifted the bedraggled black morsel. She smoothed her finger along the muddy fur and the tiny mouth opened in a soundless miaow. 'Isn't it strange? She was dying and she brought her kitten here. And on Christmas Day.'

I bent and put my hand on Debbie's heart. There was no beat.

I looked up. 'I'm afraid she's gone.' I lifted the small body, almost feather light, wrapped it in the sheet which had been spread on the rug and took it out to the car.

When I came back Mrs Ainsworth was still stroking the kitten. The tears had dried on her cheeks and she was bright-eyed as she looked at me.

'I've never had a cat before,' she said.

I smiled. 'Well it looks as though you've got one now.'

And she certainly had. That kitten grew rapidly into a sleek handsome cat with a boisterous nature which earned him the name of Buster. In every way he was the opposite to his timid little mother. Not for him the privations of the secret outdoor life; he stalked the rich carpets of the Ainsworth home like a king and the ornate collar he always wore added something more to his presence.

On my visits I watched his development with delight but the occasion which stays in my mind was the following Christmas Day, a year from his arrival.

I was out on my rounds as usual. I can't remember when I haven't had to work on Christmas Day because the animals have never got round to recognizing it as a holiday; but with the passage of the years the vague resentment I used to feel has been replaced by philosophical acceptance. After all as I tramped around the hillside barns in the frosty air I was working up a better appetite for my turkey than all the millions lying in bed or slumped by the fire; and this was aided by the innumerable aperitifs I received from the hospitable farmers.

I was on my way home, bathed in a rosy glow. I had consumed several whiskies – the kind the inexpert Yorkshiremen pour as though it was ginger ale – and I had finished with a glass of old Mrs Earnshaw's rhubarb wine which had seared its way straight to my toenails. I heard the cry as I was passing Mrs Ainsworth's house.

'Merry Christmas, Mr Herriot!' She was letting a visitor out of the front door and she waved at me gaily. 'Come in and have a drink to warm you up.'

I didn't need warming up but I pulled in to the kerb without hesitation. In the house there was all the festive cheer of last year and the same glorious whiff of sage and onion which set my gastric juices surging. But there was not the sorrow; there was Buster.

He was darting up to each of the dogs in turn, ears pricked, eyes blazing with devilment, dabbing a paw at them then streaking away.

Mrs Ainsworth laughed. 'You know, he plagues the life out of them. Gives them no peace.'

She was right. To the bassets, Buster's arrival was rather like the intrusion of an irreverent outsider into an exclusive London club. For a long time they had led a life of measured grace; regular sedate walks with their mistress, superb food in ample quantities and long snoring sessions on the rugs and armchairs. Their days followed one upon another in unruffled calm. And then came Buster.

He was dancing up to the youngest dog again, sideways

this time, head on one side, goading him. When he started boxing with both paws it was too much even for the basset. He dropped his dignity and rolled over with the cat in a brief wrestling match.

'I want to show you something.' Mrs Ainsworth lifted a hard rubber ball from the sideboard and went out to the garden, followed by Buster. She threw the ball across the lawn and the cat bounded after it over the frosted grass, the muscles rippling under the black sheen of his coat. He seized the ball in his teeth, brought it back to his mistress, dropped it at her feet and waited expectantly. She threw it and he brought it back again.

I gasped incredulously. A feline retriever!

The bassets looked on disdainfully. Nothing would ever have induced them to chase a ball, but Buster did it again and again as though he would never tire of it.

Mrs Ainsworth turned to me. 'Have you ever seen anything like that?'

'No,' I replied. 'I never have. He is a most remarkable cat.'

She snatched Buster from his play and we went back into the house where she held him close to her face, laughing as the big cat purred and arched himself ecstatically against her cheek.

Looking at him, a picture of health and contentment, my mind went back to his mother. Was it too much to think that that dying little creature with the last of her strength had carried her kitten to the only haven of comfort and warmth she had ever known in the hope that it would be cared for there? Maybe it was.

But it seemed I wasn't the only one with such fancies. Mrs Ainsworth turned to me and though she was smiling her eyes were wistful.

'Debbie would be pleased,' she said.

I nodded. 'Yes, she would . . . It was just a year ago today she brought him, wasn't it?'

'That's right.' She hugged Buster to her again. 'The best Christmas present I ever had.'

eleven

I stared in disbelief at the dial of the weighing machine. Nine stone seven pounds! I had lost two stones since joining the RAF. I was cowering in my usual corner in Boots' chemist's shop in Scarborough, where I had developed the habit of a weekly weigh-in to keep a morbid eye on my progressive emaciation. It was incredible and it wasn't all due to the tough training.

On our arrival in Scarborough we had a talk from our Flight Commander, Flt Lieut Barnes. He looked us over with a contemplative eye and said, 'You won't know yourselves when you leave here.' That man wasn't kidding.

We were never at rest. It was PT and Drill, PT and Drill, over and over. Hours of bending and stretching and twisting down on the prom in singlets and shorts while the wind whipped over us from the wintry sea. Hours of marching under the bellowings of our sergeant; quick march, slow march, about turn. We even marched to our navigation classes, bustling along at the RAF quick time, arms swinging shoulder high.

They marched us regularly to the top of Castle Hill where we fired off every conceivable type of weapon; twelve bores, ·22 rifles, revolvers, Browning machine guns. We even stabbed at dummies with bayonets. In between they had us swimming, playing football or rugby or running for miles along the beach and on the cliff tops towards Filey.

At first I was too busy to see any change in myself, but one morning after a few weeks our flight was coming to the end of a five-mile run. We dropped down from the Spa to a long stretch of empty beach and the sergeant shouted, 'Right, sprint to those rocks! Let's see who gets there first!'

We all took off on the last hundred yards' dash and I was mildly surprised to find that the first man past the post was myself – and I wasn't really out of breath. That was when the realization hit me. Mr Barnes had been right. I didn't know myself.

When I left Helen I was a cosseted young husband with a little double chin and the beginnings of a spare tyre, and now I was a lithe, tireless greyhound. I was certainly fit, but there was something wrong. I shouldn't have been as thin as this. Another factor was at work.

In Yorkshire when a man goes into a decline during his wife's pregnancy they giggle behind their hands and say he is 'carrying' the baby. I never laugh at these remarks because I am convinced I 'carried' my son.

I base this conclusion on a variety of symptoms. It would be an exaggeration to say I suffered from morning sickness, but my suspicions were certainly aroused when I began to feel a little queasy in the early part of the day. This was followed by a growing uneasiness as Helen's time drew near and a sensation, despite my physical condition, of being drained and miserable. With the onset in the later stages of unmistakable labour pains in my lower abdomen all doubts were resolved and I knew I had to do something about it.

I had to see Helen. After all, she was just over that hill which I could see from the top windows of the Grand. Maybe that wasn't strictly true, but at least I was in Yorkshire and a bus would take me to her in three hours. The snag was that there was no leave from ITW. They left us in no doubt about that. They said the discipline was as tough as a Guards regiment and the restrictions just as rigid. I would get compassionate leave when the baby was born, but I couldn't wait till then. The grim knowledge that any attempt to dodge off unofficially would be like a minor desertion and would be followed by serious consequences, even prison, didn't weigh with me.

As one of my comrades put it: 'One bloke tried it and finished up in the Glasshouse. It isn't worth it, mate.'

But it was no good. I am normally a law-abiding citizen but I had not a single scruple. I had to see Helen. A surreptitious study of the timetables revealed that there was a bus at 2 p.m. which got to Darrowby at five o'clock, and another leaving Darrowby at six which arrived in Scarborough at nine. Six hours travelling to have one hour with Helen. It was worth it.

At first I couldn't see a way of getting to the bus station at two o'clock in the afternoon because we were never free at that time, but my chance came quite unexpectedly. One Friday lunchtime we learned that there were no more classes that day but we were confined to the Grand till evening. Most of my friends collapsed thankfully on to their beds, but I slunk down the long flights of stone stairs and took up a position in the foyer where I could watch the front door.

There was a glass-fronted office on one side of the entrance where the SPs sat and kept an eye on all departures. There was only one on duty today and I waited till he turned and moved to the back of the room then I walked quietly past him and out into the square.

That part had been almost too easy, but I felt naked and exposed as I crossed the deserted space between the Grand and the hotels on the opposite side. It was better once I had rounded the corner and I set off at a brisk pace for the west. All I needed was a little bit of luck and as I pressed, dry-mouthed, along the empty street it seemed I had found it. The shock when I saw the two burly SPs strolling towards me was like a blow but was immediately followed by a strange calm.

They would ask me for the pass I didn't have, then they would want to know what I was doing there. It wouldn't be much good telling them I had just popped out for a breath of air – this street led to both the bus and railway stations and it wouldn't need a genius to rumble my little game. Anyway, there was no cover here, no escape, and I wondered idly if there had ever been a veterinary surgeon in the Glasshouse. Maybe I was about to set up some kind of a record.

Then behind me I heard the rhythmic tramp of marching feet and the shrill ''eft 'ight, 'eft 'ight,' that usually went with it. I turned and saw a long blue column approaching with a corporal in charge. As they swung past me I looked again at the SPs and my hear gave a thud. They were laughing into each other's faces at some private joke; they hadn't seen me. Without thinking I tagged on to the end of the marching men and within a few seconds was past the SPs unnoticed.

With my mind working with the speed of desperation, it seemed I would be safest where I was till I could break away in the direction of the bus station. For a while I had a glorious feeling of anonymity, then the corporal, still shouting, glanced back. He faced to the front again then turned back more slowly for another look. He appeared to find something interesting because he shortened his stride till he was marching opposite me.

As he looked me up and down I examined him in turn from the corner of my eye. He was a shrivelled, runtish creature with fierce little eyes glinting from a pallid, skull-like face. It was some time before he spoke.

'Who the — hell are you?' he enquired conversationally. It was the number one awkward question but I discerned the faintest gleam of hope; he had spoken in the unmistakable harsh, glottal accent of my home town.

'Herriot, corporal. Two flight, four squadron,' I replied in my broadest Glasgow.

'Two flight, four . . . ! This is one flight, three squadron. What the — hell are ye daein' here?'

Arms swinging high, staring rigidly ahead, I took a deep breath. Concealment was futile now.

'Tryin' to get tae see ma wife, corp. She's havin' a baby soon.'

I glanced quickly at him. His was not the kind of face to reveal weakness by showing surprise but his eyes widened fractionally. 'Get tae see yer wife? Are ye — daft or whit?'

'It's no' far, corp. She lives in Darrowby. Three hours in the bus. Ah wid be back tonight.'

'Back tonight! Ye want yer — heid examinin'!'

'I've got tae go!'

'Eyes front!' he screamed suddenly at the men before us. ''eft 'ight, 'eft 'ight!' Then he turned and studied me as though I were an unbelievable phenomenon. He was interesting to me, too, as a typical product of the bad times in Glasgow between the wars. Stunted, undernourished, but as tough and belligerent as a ferret.

'D'ye no' ken,' he said at length, 'that ye get — leave when yer wife has the wean?'

'Aye, but ah canna' wait that long. Gimme a break, corp.'

'Give ye a — break! D'ye want tae get me — shot?'

'No, corp, just want tae get to the bus station.'

'Jesus! Is that a'?' He gave me a final incredulous look before quickening his steps to the head of the column. When he returned he surveyed me again.

'Whit part o' Glesca are ye frae?'

'Scotstounhill,' I replied. 'How about you?'

'Govan.'

I turned my head slightly towards him. 'Rangers supporter, eh?'

He did not change expression, but an eyebrow flickered and I knew I had him.

'Whit a team!' I murmured reverently. 'Many's the time I've stood on the terraces at Ibrox.'

He said nothing and I began to recite the names of the great Rangers team of the thirties. 'Dawson, Gray, McDonald, Meiklejohn, Simpson, Brown.' His eyes took on a dreamy expression and by the time I had intoned 'Archibald, Marshall, English, McPhail and Morton,' there was something near to a wistful smile on his lips.

Then he appeared to shake himself back to normality.

''Eft 'ight, 'eft 'ight!' he bawled. 'C'mon, c'mon, pick it up!' Then he muttered to me from the corner of his mouth. 'There's the — bus station. When we march past it run like — !'

He took off again, shouting to the head of the flight, I saw the buses and the windows of the waiting room on my left and dived across the road and through the door. I snatched off my cap and sat trembling among a group of elderly farmers and their wives. Through the glass I could see the long lines of blue moving away down the street and I could still hear the shouts of the corporal.

But he didn't turn round and I saw only his receding back, the narrow shoulders squared, the bent legs stepping it out in time with his men. I never saw him again but to this day I wish I could take him to Ibrox and watch the Rangers with him and maybe buy him a half and half pint at one of the Govan pubs. It wouldn't have mattered if he had turned out to be a Celtic supporter at that decisive moment because I had the Celtic team on my tongue all ready to trot out, starting with Kennaway, Cook, McGonigle. It is not the only time my profound knowledge of football has stood me in good stead.

Sitting on the bus, still with my cap on my lap to avoid attracting attention, it struck me that the whole world changed within a mile or two as we left the town. Back there the war was everywhere, filling people's minds and eyes and thoughts; the teeming thousands of uniformed men, the RAF and army vehicles, the almost palpable atmosphere of anticipation and suspense. And suddenly it all just stopped.

It vanished as the wide sweep of grey-blue sea fell beneath the rising ground behind the town, and as the bus trundled westward I looked out on a landscape of untroubled peace. The long moist furrows of the new-turned soil glittered under the pale February sun, contrasting with the gold stubble fields and the grassy pastures where sheep clustered around their feeding troughs. There was no wind and the smoke rose straight from the farm chimneys and the bare branches of the roadside trees were still as they stretched across the cold sky.

There were many things that pulled at me. A man in breeches and leggings carrying on his shoulder a bale of hay to some outlying cattle; a group of farm men burning hedge clippings and the fragrance of the wood smoke finding its way into the bus. The pull was stronger as the hours passed and the beginnings of my own familiar countryside began to appear beyond the windows. Maybe it was a good thing I didn't see Darrowby; Helen's home was near the bus route and I dropped off well short of the town.

She was alone in the house and she turned her head as I walked into the kitchen. The delight on her face was mixed with astonishment; in fact I know we were both astonished, she because I was so skinny and I because she was so fat. Helen, with the baby only two weeks away, was very large indeed, but not too large for me to get my arms around her, and we stood there in the middle of the flagged floor clasped together for a long time with neither of us saying much.

She cooked me egg and chips and sat by me while I ate. We carried on a rather halting conversation and it came to me with a bump that my mind had been forced on to different tracks since I had left her. In those few months my brain had become saturated with the things of my new life – even my mouth was full of RAF slang and jargon. In our bed-sitter we used to talk about my cases, the funny things that happened on my rounds, but now, I thought helplessly, there wasn't much point in telling her that AC2 Phillips was on jankers again, that vector triangles were the very devil, that Don McGregor thought he had discovered the secret of Sergeant Hynd's phenomenally shiny boots.

But it really didn't matter. My worries melted as I looked at her. I had been wondering if she was well and there she was, bouncing with energy, shining-eyed, rosy-cheeked and beautiful. There was only one jarring note and it was a strange one. Helen was wearing a 'maternity dress' which expanded with the passage of time by means of an opening down one side. Anyway, I hated it. It was blue with a high red collar and I thought it cheap-looking and ugly. I was aware that austerity had taken over in England and that a lot of things were shoddy, but I desperately wished my wife had something better to wear. In all my life there have been very few occasions when I badly wanted more money and that was one of them, because on my wage of three shillings a day as an AC2 I was unable to drape her with expensive clothes.

The hour winged past and it seemed no time at all before I was back on the top road waiting in the gathering darkness for the Scarborough bus. The journey back was a bit dreary as the blacked-out vehicle bumped and rattled its way through the darkened villages and over the long stretches of anonymous countryside. It was cold, too, but I sat there happily with the memory of Helen wrapped around me like a warm quilt.

The whole day had been a triumph. I had got away by a lucky stroke and there would be no problem getting back into the Grand because one of my pals would be on sentry duty and it would be a case of 'pass friend'. Closing my eyes in the gloom I could still feel Helen in my arms and I smiled to myself at the memory of her bounding healthiness. She looked marvellous, the egg and chips tasted wonderful, everything was great.

Except that one discord which jangled still. Oh, how I hated that dress!

twelve

'Hey you! Where the 'ell d'you think you're goin'?'

Coming from the RAF Special Police it was a typical mode of address and the man who barked it out wore the usual truculent expression.

'Extra navigation class, corporal,' I replied.

'Lemme see your pass!'

He snatched it from my hand, read it and returned it without looking at me. I slunk out into the street feeling like a prisoner on parole.

Not all the SPs were like that but I found most of them lacking in charm. And it brought home to me with a rush something which had been slowly dawning on me ever since I joined the Air Force; that I had been spoiled for quite a long time now. Spoiled by the fact that I had always been treated with respect because I was a veterinary surgeon, a member of an honourable profession. And I had taken it entirely for granted.

Now I was an AC2, the lowest form of life in the RAF, and the 'Hey you!' was a reflection of my status. The Yorkshire farmers don't rush out and kiss you, but their careful friendliness and politeness is something which I have valued even more since my service days. Because that was when I stopped taking it for granted.

Mind you, you have to put up with a certain amount of

cheek in most jobs, and veterinary practice is no exception. Even now I can recall the glowering face of Ralph Beamish the racehorse trainer, as he watched me getting out of my car.

'Where's Mr Farnon?' he grunted.

My toes curled. I had heard that often enough, especially among the horse fraternity around Darrowby.

'I'm sorry, Mr Beamish, but he'll be away all day and I thought I'd better come along rather than leave it till tomorrow.'

He made no attempt to hide his disgust. He blew out his fat, purpled cheeks, dug his hands deep in his breeches pockets and looked at the sky with a martyred air.

'Well come on, then.' He turned and stumped away on his short, thick legs towards one of the boxes which bordered the yard. I sighed inwardly as I followed him. Being an unhorsey vet in Yorkshire was a penance at times, especially in a racing stable like this which was an equine shrine. Siegfried, apart altogether from his intuitive skill, was able to talk the horse language. He could discuss effortlessly and at length the breeding and points of his patients; he rode, he hunted, he even looked the part with his long aristocratic face, clipped moustache and lean frame.

The trainers loved him and some, like Beamish, took it as a mortal insult when he failed to come in person to minister to their valuable charges.

He called to one of the lads who opened a box door.

'He's in there,' he muttered. 'Came in lame from exercise this morning.'

The lad led out a bay gelding and there was no need to trot the animal to diagnose the affected leg; he nodded down on his near fore in an unmistakable way.

'I think he's lame in the shoulder,' Beamish said.

I went round the other side of the horse and picked up the off fore. I cleaned out the frog and sole with a hoof knife; there was no sign of bruising and no sensitivity when I tapped the handle of the knife against the horn.

I felt my way over the coronet to the fetlock and after

some palpation I located a spot near the distal end of the metacarpus which was painful on pressure.

I looked up from my crouching position. 'This seems to be the trouble, Mr Beamish. I think he must have struck into himself with his hind foot just there.'

'Where?' The trainer leaned over me and peered down at the leg. 'I can't see anything.'

'No, the skin isn't broken, but he flinches if you press here.'

Beamish prodded the place with a stubby forefinger.

'Well, he does,' he grunted. 'But he'd flinch anywhere if you squeeze him like you're doing.'

My hackles began to rise at his tone but I kept my voice calm. 'I'm sure that's what it is. I should apply a hot anti-phlogistine poultice just above the fetlock and alternate with a cold hose on it twice a day.'

'Well, I'm just as sure you're wrong. It's not down there at all. The way that horse carries his leg he's hurt his shoulder.' He gestured to the lad. 'Harry, see that he gets some heat on that shoulder right away.'

If the man had struck me I couldn't have felt worse. I opened my mouth to argue but he was walking away.

'There's another horse I want you to look at,' he said. He led the way into a nearby box and pointed to a big brown animal with obvious signs of blistering on the tendons of a fore limb.

'Mr Farnon put a red blister on that leg six months ago. He's been resting in here ever since. He's going sound now – d'you think he's ready to go out?'

I went over and ran my fingers over the length of the flexor tendons, feeling for signs of thickening. There was none. Then I lifted the foot and as I explored further I found a tender area in the superficial flexor.

I straightened up. 'He's still a bit sore,' I said. 'I think it would be safer to keep him in for a bit longer.'

'Can't agree with you,' Beamish snapped. He turned to the lad. 'Turn him out, Harry.'

I stared at him. Was this a deliberate campaign to make me

feel small? Was he trying to rub in the fact that he didn't think much of me? Anyway, he was beginning to get under my skin and I hoped my burning face wasn't too obvious.

'One thing more,' Beamish said. 'There's a horse through here been coughing. Have a look at him before you go.'

We went through a narrow passage into a smaller yard and Harry entered a box and got hold of a horse's head collar. I followed him, fishing out my thermometer.

As I approached the animal's rear end he laid back his ears, whickered and began to caper around. I hesitated, then nodded to the lad.

'Lift his fore leg while I take his temperature, will you?' I said.

The lad bent down and seized the foot but Beamish broke in. 'Don't bother, Harry, there's no need for that. He's quiet as a sheep.'

I paused for a moment. I felt I was right but my stock was low on this establishment. I shrugged, lifted the tail and pushed the thermometer into the rectum.

The two hind feet hit me almost simultaneously but as I sailed backwards through the door I remember thinking quite clearly that the one on the chest had made contact fractionally before the one on the abdomen. But my thoughts were rapidly clouded by the fact that the lower hoof had landed full on my solar plexus.

Stretched on the concrete of the yard I gasped and groaned in a frantic search for breath. There was a moment when I was convinced I was going to die but at last a long wailing respiration came to my aid and I struggled painfully into a sitting position. Through the open door I could see Harry hanging on to the horse's head and staring at me with frightened eyes. Mr Beamish, on the other hand, showed no interest in my plight; he was anxiously examining the horse's hind feet one after the other. Obviously he was worried lest they may have sustained some damage by coming into contact with my nasty hard ribs.

Slowly I got up and drew some long breaths. I was shaken but not really hurt. And I suppose it was instinct that had made me hang on to my thermometer; the delicate tube was still in my hand.

My only emotion as I went back into the box was cold rage.

'Lift that bloody foot like I told you!' I shouted at the unfortunate Harry.

'Right, sir! Sorry, sir!' He bent, lifted the foot and held it cupped firmly in his hands.

I turned to Beamish to see if he had any observation to make, but the trainer was silent, gazing at the big animal expressionlessly.

This time I took the temperature without incident. It was 101°F. I moved to the head and opened the nostril with finger and thumb, revealing a slight muco-purulent discharge. Sub-maxillary and post-pharyngeal glands were normal.

'He's got a bit of a cold,' I said. 'I'll give him an injection and leave you some sulphonamide – that's what Mr Farnon uses in these cases.' If my final sentence reassured him in any way he gave no sign, watching dead-faced as I injected 10 cc of Prontosil.

Before I left I took a half-pound packet of sulphonamide from the car boot. 'Give him three ounces of this immediately in a pint of water, then follow it with one and a half ounces night and morning and let us know if he isn't a lot better in two days.'

Mr Beamish received the medicine unsmilingly and as I opened the car door I felt a gush of relief that the uncomfortable visit was at an end. It seemed to have lasted a long time and there had been no glory for me in it. I was starting the engine when one of the little apprentices panted up to the trainer.

'It's Almira, sir. I think she's chokin'!'

'Choking!' Beamish stared at the boy then whipped round to me. 'Almira's the best filly I have. You'd better come!'

It wasn't over yet, then. With a feeling of doom I hurried after the squat figure back into the yard where another lad stood by the side of a beautiful chestnut filly. And as I saw her a cold hand closed around my heart. I had been dealing with trivia but this was different.

She stood immobile, staring ahead with a peculiar intensity. The rise and fall of her ribs was accompanied by a rasping, bubbling wheeze and at each intake her nostrils flared wildly. I had never seen a horse breathe like this. And there were other things; saliva drooled from her lips and every few seconds she gave a retching cough.

I turned to the apprentice. 'When did this start?'

'Not long ago, sir. I saw her an hour since and she were as right as a bobbin.'

'Are you sure?'

'Aye, I was givin' 'er some hay. There was nowt ailin' her then.'

'What the devil's wrong with her?' Beamish exclaimed.

Well, it was a good question and I didn't have a clue to the answer. As I walked bemusedly round the animal, taking in the trembling limbs and terrified eyes, a jumble of thoughts crowded my brain. I had seen 'choking' horses – the dry choke when the gullet becomes impacted with food – but they didn't look like this. I felt my way along the course of the oesophagus and it was perfectly clear. And anyway the respiration was quite different. This filly looked as though she had some obstruction in her airflow. But what . . . ? And how . . . ? Could there be a foreign body in there? Just possible, but that was something else I had never seen.

'Well, damn it, I'm asking you! What is it? What d'you make of her?' Mr Beamish was becoming impatient and I couldn't blame him.

I was aware that I was slightly breathless. 'Just a moment while I listen to her lungs.'

'Just a moment!' the trainer burst out. 'Good God, man, we haven't got many moments! This horse could die!'

He didn't have to tell me. I had seen that ominous trembling of the limbs before and now the filly was beginning to sway a little. Time was running out.

Dry mouthed, I auscultated the chest. I knew there was nothing wrong with her lungs – the trouble seemed to be in the throat area – but it gave me a little more time to think. Even with the stethoscope in my ears I could still hear Beamish's voice.

'It would have to be this one! Sir Eric Horrocks gave five thousand pounds for her last year. She's the most valuable animal in my stables. Why did this have to happen?'

Groping my way over the ribs, my heart thudding, I heartily agreed with him. Why in heaven's name did I have to walk into this nightmare? And with a man like Beamish who had no faith in me.

He stepped forward and clutched my arm. 'Are you sure Mr Farnon isn't available?'

'I'm sorry,' I replied huskily. 'He's over thirty miles away.'

The trainer seemed to shrivel within himself. 'That's it then. We're finished. She's dying.'

And he was right. The filly had begun to reel about, the breathing louder and more stertorous than ever, and I had difficulty in keeping the stethoscope on her chest wall. It was when I was resting my hand on her flank to steady her that I noticed the little swelling under the skin. It was a circular plaque, like a penny pushed under the tissue. I glanced sharply at it. Yes, it was clearly visible. And there was another one higher up on the back ... and another and another. My heart gave a quick double thump ... so that was it.

'What am I going to tell Sir Eric?' the trainer groaned. 'That his filly is dead and the vet didn't know what was wrong with her?' He glared desperately around him as though in the faint hope that Siegfried might magically appear from nowhere.

I called over my shoulder as I trotted towards the car. 'I never said I didn't know. I do know. She's got urticaria.'

He came shambling after me. 'Urti ... what the blazes is that?'

'Nettlerash,' I replied, fumbling among my bottles for the adrenalin.

'Nettlerash!' His eyes widened. 'But that couldn't cause all this!'

I drew 5 cc of the adrenalin into the syringe and started back. 'It's nothing to do with nettles. It's an allergic condition, usually pretty harmless, but in a very few cases it causes oedema of the larynx – that's what we've got here.'

It was difficult to raise the vein as the filly staggered around, but she came to rest for a few seconds and I dug my thumb into the jugular furrow. As the big vessel came up tense and turgid I thrust in the needle and injected the adrenalin. Then I stepped back and stood by the trainer's side.

Neither of us said anything. The spectacle of the toiling animal and the harrowing sound of the breathing absorbed us utterly.

The grim knowledge that she was on the verge of suffocation appalled me and when she stumbled and almost fell the hand in my pocket gripped more tightly on the scalpel which I had taken from my car along with the adrenalin. I knew only too well that tracheotomy was indicated here but I didn't have a tube with me. If the filly did go off her legs I should have to start cutting into her windpipe, but I put the thought away from me. For the moment I had to depend on the adrenalin.

Beamish stretched out a hand in a helpless gesture. 'It's hopeless, isn't it?' he whispered.

I shrugged. 'There's a small chance. If the injection can reduce the fluid in the larynx in time . . . we'll just have to wait.'

He nodded and I could read more than one emotion in his face; not just the dread of breaking the news to the famous owner but the distress of a horse-lover as he witnessed the plight of the beautiful animal.

At first I thought it was imagination, but it seemed that the breathing was becoming less stertorous. Then as I hovered in an agony of uncertainty I noticed that the salivation was diminishing; she was able to swallow.

From that moment events moved with unbelievable rapidity. The symptoms of allergies appear with dramatic suddenness but mercifully they often disappear as quickly following treatment. Within fifteen minutes the filly looked almost normal. There was still a slight wheeze in her respirations but she was looking around her, quite free from distress.

Beamish, who had been watching like a man in a daze, pulled a handful of hay from a bale and held it out to her. She snatched it eagerly from his hand and began to eat with great relish.

'I can't believe it,' the trainer muttered almost to himself. 'I've never seen anything work as fast as that injection.'

I felt as though I was riding on a pink cloud with all the tension and misery flowing from me in a joyful torrent. Thank God there were moments like this among the traumas of veterinary work; the sudden transition from despair to triumph, from shame to pride.

I almost floated to the car and as I settled in my seat Beamish put his face to the open window.

'Mr Herriot . . .' He was not a man to whom gracious speech came easily and his cheeks, roughened and weathered by years of riding on the open moor, twitched as he sought for words. 'Mr Herriot, I've been thinking . . . you don't have to be a horsey man to cure horses, do you?'

There was something like an appeal in his eyes as we gazed at each other. I laughed suddenly and his expression relaxed.

'That's right,' I said, and drove away.

thirteen

Do dogs have a sense of humour?

I felt I needed all mine as I stood on guard outside the Grand. It was after midnight, with a biting wind swirling across the empty square, and I was so cold and bored that it was a relief even to slap the butt of my rifle in salute as a solitary officer went by.

Wryly I wondered how, after my romantic ideas of training to be a pilot, I came to be defending the Grand Hotel at Scarborough against all comers. No doubt there was something comic in the situation and I suppose that was what set my mind wandering in the direction of Farmer Bailes' dog, Shep.

Mr Bailes' little place was situated about half way along Highburn village and to get into the farmyard you had to walk twenty yards or so between five-foot walls. On the left was the neighbouring house, on the right the front garden of the farm. In this garden Shep lurked for most of the day.

He was a huge dog, much larger than the average collie. In fact I am convinced he was part Alsatian because though he had a luxuriant black and white coat there was something significant in the massive limbs and in the noble brown-shaded head with its upstanding ears. He was quite different from the stringy little animals I saw on my daily round.

As I walked between the walls my mind was already in the byre, just visible at the far end of the yard. Because one of the Bailes cows, Rose by name, had the kind of obscure digestive ailment which interferes with veterinary surgeons' sleep. They are so difficult to diagnose. This animal had begun to grunt and go off her milk two days ago and when I had seen her yesterday I had flitted from one possibility to the other. Could be a wire. But the fourth stomach was contracting well and there were plenty of rumenal sounds. Also she was eating a little hay in a half-hearted way.

Could it be impaction . . . ? Or a partial torsion of the gut . . . ? There was abdominal pain without a doubt and that nagging temperature of 102·5° – that was damn like a wire. Of course I could settle the whole thing by opening the cow up, but Mr Bailes was an old-fashioned type and didn't like the idea of my diving into his animal unless I was certain of my diagnosis. And I wasn't – there was no getting away from that.

Anyway, I had built her up at the front end so that she was standing with her fore feet on a half door and had given her a strong oily purgative. 'Keep the bowels open and trust in

God,' an elderly colleague had once told me. There was a lot in that.

I was half way down the alley between the walls with the hope bright before me that my patient would be improved when from nowhere an appalling explosion of sound blasted into my right ear. It was Shep again.

The wall was just the right height for the dog to make a leap and bark into the ear of the passers by. It was a favourite gambit of his and I had been caught before; but never so successfully as now. My attention had been so far away and the dog had timed his jump to a split second so that his bark came at the highest point, his teeth only inches from my face. And his voice befitted his size, a great bull bellow surging from the depths of his powerful chest and booming from his gaping jaws.

I rose several inches into the air and when I descended, heart thumping, head singing, I glared over the wall. But as usual all I saw was the hairy form bounding away out of sight round the corner of the house.

That was what puzzled me. Why did he do it? Was he a savage creature with evil designs on me or was it his idea of a joke? I never got near enough to him to find out.

I wasn't in the best of shape to receive bad news and that was what awaited me in the byre. I had only to look at the farmer's face to know that the cow was worse.

'Ah reckon she's got a stoppage,' Mr Bailes muttered gloomily.

I gritted my teeth. The entire spectrum of abdominal disorders were lumped as 'stoppages' by the older race of farmers. 'The oil hasn't worked, then?'

'Nay, she's nobbut passin' little hard bits. It's a proper stoppage, ah tell you.'

'Right, Mr Bailes,' I said with a twisted smile. 'We'll have to try something stronger.' I brought in from my car the gastric lavage outfit I loved so well and which has so sadly disappeared from my life. The long rubber stomach tube, the wooden gag with its leather straps to buckle behind the horns. As I pumped in the two gallons of warm water rich in formalin and sodium chloride I felt like Napoleon sending in the Old Guard at Waterloo. If this didn't work nothing would.

And yet I didn't feel my usual confidence. There was something different here. But I had to try. I had to do something to start this cow's insides functioning because I did not like the look of her today. The soft grunt was still there and her eyes had begun to retreat into her head – the worst sign of all in bovines. And she had stopped eating altogether.

Next morning I was driving down the single village street when I saw Mrs Bailes coming out of the shop. I drew up and pushed my head out of the window.

'How's Rose this morning, Mrs Bailes?'

She rested her basket on the ground and looked down at me gravely. 'Oh, she's bad, Mr Herriot. Me husband thinks she's goin' down fast. If you want to find him you'll have to go across the field there. He's mendin' the door in that little barn.'

A sudden misery enveloped me as I drove over to the gate leading into the field. I left the car in the road and lifted the latch.

'Damn! Damn! Damn!' I muttered as I trailed across the green. I had a nasty feeling that a little tragedy was building up here. If this animal died it would be a sickening blow to a small farmer with ten cows and a few pigs. I should be able to do something about it and it was a depressing thought that I was getting nowhere.

And yet, despite it all, I felt peace stealing into my soul. It was a large field and I could see the barn at the far end as I walked with the tall grass brushing my knees. It was a meadow ready for cutting and suddenly I realized that it was high summer, the sun was hot and that every step brought the fragrance of clover and warm grass rising about me into the crystal freshness of the air. Somewhere nearby a field of broad beans was in full flower and as the exotic scent drifted across I found myself inhaling with half-closed eyes as though straining to discern the ingredients of the glorious melange.

And then there was the silence; it was the most soothing thing of all. That and the feeling of being alone. I looked drowsily around at the empty green miles sleeping under the sunshine. Nothing stirred, there was no sound.

Then without warning the ground at my feet erupted in an incredible blast of noise. For a dreadful moment the blue sky was obscured by an enormous hairy form and a red mouth went 'WAAAHH!' in my face. Almost screaming, I staggered back and as I glared wildly I saw Shep disappearing at top speed towards the gate. Concealed in the deep herbage right in the middle of the field he had waited till he saw the whites of my eyes before making his assault.

Whether he had been there by accident or whether he had spotted me arriving and slunk into position I shall never know, but from his point of view the result must have been eminently satisfactory because it was certainly the worst fright I have ever had. I live a life which is well larded with scares and alarms, but this great dog rising bellowing from that empty landscape was something on its own. I have heard of cases where sudden terror and stress has caused involuntary evacuation of the bowels and I know without question that this was the occasion when I came nearest to suffering that unhappy fate.

I was still trembling when I reached the barn and hardly said a word as Mr Bailes led me back across the road to the farm.

And it was like rubbing it in when I saw my patient. The flesh had melted from her and she stared at the wall apathetically from sunken eyes. The doom-laden grunt was louder.

'She must have a wire!' I muttered. 'Let her loose for a minute, will you?'

Mr Bailes undid the chain and Rose walked along the byre. At the end she turned and almost trotted back to her stall, jumping quite freely over the gutter. My Bible in those days was Udall's *Practice of Veterinary Medicine* and the great man stated therein that if a cow moved freely she was unlikely to have a foreign body in her reticulum. I pinched her withers and she didn't complain . . . it had to be something else.

'It's worst stoppage ah've seen for a bit,' said Mr Bailes. 'Ah gave her a dose of some right powerful stuff this mornin' but it's done no good.'

I passed a weary hand over my brow. 'What was that, Mr Bailes?' It was always a bad sign when the client started using his own medicine.

The farmer reached to the cluttered windowsill and handed me a bottle. 'Doctor Hornibrook's Stomach Elixir. A sovereign remedy for all diseases of cattle.' The Doctor, in top hat and frock coat, looked confidently out at me from the label as I pulled out the cork and took a sniff. I blinked and staggered back with watering eyes. It smelt like pure ammonia but I was in no position to be superior about it.

'That dang grunt!' The farmer hunched his shoulders. 'What's cause of it?'

It was no good my saying it sounded like a circumscribed area of peritonitis because I didn't know what was behind it.

I decided to have one last go with the lavage. It was still the strongest weapon in my armoury but this time I added two pounds of black treacle to the mixture. Nearly every farmer had a barrel of the stuff in his cow house in those days and I had only to go into the corner and turn the tap.

I often mourn the passing of the treacle barrel because molasses was a good medicine for cattle, but I had no great hopes this time. The clinical instinct I was beginning to develop told me that something inside this animal was fundamentally awry.

It was not till the following afternoon that I drove into Highburn. I left the car outside the farm and was about to walk between the walls when I paused and stared at a cow in the field on the other side of the road. It was a pasture next to the hayfield of yesterday and that cow was Rose. There could be no mistake – she was a fine deep red with a distinctive white mark like a football on her left flank.

I opened the gate and within seconds my cares dropped from me. She was wonderfully, miraculously improved, in fact she looked like a normal animal. I walked up to her and scratched the root of her tail. She was a docile creature and merely looked round at me as she cropped the grass; and her eyes were no longer sunken but bright and full.

She seemed to take a fancy to a green patch further into the field and began to amble slowly towards it. I followed, entranced, as she moved along, shaking her head impatiently against the flies, eager for more of the delicious herbage. The grunt had disappeared and her udder hung heavy and turgid between her legs. The difference since yesterday was incredible.

As the wave of relief flooded through me I saw Mr Bailes climbing over the wall from the next field. He would still be mending that barn door.

As he approached I felt apang of commiseration. I had to guard against any display of triumph. He must be feeling just a bit silly at the moment after showing his lack of faith in me yesterday with his home remedies and his general attitude. But after all the poor chap had been worried – I couldn't blame him. No, it wouldn't do to preen myself unduly.

'Ah, good morning to you, Mr Bailes,' I said expansively. 'Rose looks fine today, doesn't she?'

The farmer took off his cap and wiped his brow. 'Aye, she's a different cow, all right.'

'I don't think she needs any more treatment,' I said. I hesitated. Perhaps one little dig would do no harm. 'But it's a good thing I gave her that extra lavage yesterday.'

'Yon pumpin' job?' Mr Bailes raised his eyebrows. 'Oh that had nowt to do with it.'

'What . . . what do you mean? It cured her, surely.'

'Nay, lad, nay, Jim Oakley cured her.'

'Jim . . . what on earth . . . ?'

'Aye, Jim was round 'ere last night. He often comes in of an evenin' and he took one look at the cow and told me what to do. Ah'll tell you she was like dyin' – that pumpin' job hadn't done no good at all. He told me to give her a bloody good gallop round t'field.'

'What!'

'Aye, that's what he said. He'd seen 'em like that afore and

116

a good gallop put 'em right. So we got Rose out here and did as he said and by gaw it did the trick. She looked better right away.'

I drew myself up. 'And who,' I asked frigidly, 'is Jim Oakley?'

'He's t'postman, of course.'

'The postman!'

'Aye, but he used to keep a few beasts years ago. He's a very clever man wi' stock, is Jim.'

'No doubt, but I assure you, Mr Bailes . . .'

The farmer raised a hand. 'Say no more, lad. Jim put 'er right and there's no denyin' it. I wish you'd seen 'im chasin' 'er round. He's as awd as me, but by gaw 'e did go. He can run like'ell, can Jim.' He chuckled reminiscently.

I had had about enough. During the farmer's eulogy I had been distractedly scratching the cow's tail and had soiled my hand in the process. Mustering the remains of my dignity I nodded to Mr Bailes.

'Well, I must be on my way. Do you mind if I go into the house to wash my hands?'

'You go right in,' he replied. 'T'missus will get you some hot water.'

Walking back down the field the cruel injustice of the thing bore down on me increasingly. I wandered as in a dream through the gate and across road. Before entering the alley between the walls I glanced into the garden. It was empty. Shuffling beside the rough stones I sank deeper into my misery. There was no doubt I had emerged from that episode as a complete Charlie. No matter where I looked I couldn't see a gleam of light.

It seemed to take a long time to reach the end of the wall and I was about to turn right towards the door of the farm kitchen when from my left I heard the sudden rattle of a chain then a roaring creature launched itself at me, bayed once, mightily, into my face and was gone.

This time I thought my heart would stop. With my defences at their lowest I was in no state to withstand Shep. I had quite forgotten that Mrs Bailes occasionally tethered him in the kennel at the entrance to discourage unwelcome visitors, and as I half lay against the wall, the blood thundering in my ears, I looked dully at the long coil of chain on the cobbles.

I have no time for people who lose their temper with animals but something snapped in my mind then. All my frustration burst from me in a torrent of incoherent shouts and I grabbed the chain and began to pull on it frenziedly. That dog which had tortured me was there in that kennel. For once I knew where to get at him and this time I was going to have the matter out with him. The kennel would be about ten feet away and at first I saw nothing. There was only the dead weight on the end of the chain. Then as I hauled inexorably a nose appeared, then a head, then all of the big animal hanging limply by his collar. He showed no desire to get up and greet me but I was merciless and dragged him inch by inch over the cobbles till he was lying at my feet.

Beside myself with rage, I crouched, shook my fist under his nose and yelled at him from a few inches' range.

'You big bugger! If you do that to me again I'll knock your bloody head off! Do you hear me, I'll knock your bloody head clean off!'

Shep rolled frightened eyes at me and his tail flickered apologetically between his legs. When I continued to scream at him he bared his upper teeth in an ingratiating grin and finally rolled on his back where he lay inert with half-closed eyes.

So now I knew. He was a softie. All his ferocious attacks were just a game. I began to calm down but for all that I wanted him to get the message.

'Right, mate,' I said in a menacing whisper. 'Remember what I've said!' I let go the chain and gave a final shout. 'Now get back in there!'

Shep, almost on his knees, tail tucked well in, shot back into his kennel and I turned toward the farmhouse to wash my hands.

The memory of my discomfiture fermented in the back of

my mind for some time. I had no doubt then that I had been unfairly judged, but I am older and wiser now and in retrospect I think I was wrong.

The symptoms displayed by Mr Bailes' cow were typical of displacement of the abomasum (when the fourth stomach slips round from the right to the left side) and it was a condition that was just not recognized in those early days.

At the present time we correct the condition by surgery – pushing the displaced organ back to the right side and tacking it there with sutures. But sometimes a similar result can be obtained by casting the cow and rolling her over, so why not by making her run . . . ? I freely admit that I have many times adopted Jim Oakley's precept of a 'bloody good gallop', often with spectacular results. To this day I frequently learn things from farmers, but that was one time when I learned from a postman.

I was surprised when, about a month later, I received another call to one of Mr Bailes' cows. I felt that after my performance with Rose he would have called on the services of Jim Oakley for any further trouble. But no, his voice on the phone was as polite and friendly as ever, with not a hint that he had lost faith. It was strange. . . .

Leaving my car outside the farm I looked warily into the front garden before venturing between the walls. A faint tinkle of metal told me that Shep was lurking there in his kennel and I slowed my steps; I wasn't going to be caught again. At the end of the alley I paused, waiting, but all I saw was the end of a nose which quietly withdrew as I stood there. So my outburst had got through to the big dog – he knew I wasn't going to stand any more nonsense from him.

And yet, as I drove away after the visit I didn't feel good about it. A victory over an animal is a hollow one and I had the uncomfortable feeling that I had deprived him of his chief pleasure. After all, every creature is entitled to some form of recreation and though Shep's hobby could result in the occasional heart failure it was, after all, his thing and part of him. The thought that I had crushed something out of his life was a disquieting one. I wasn't proud.

So that when, later that summer, I was driving through Highburn I paused in anticipation outside the Bailes farm. The village street, white and dusty, slumbered under the afternoon sun. In the blanketing silence nothing moved – except for one small man strolling towards the opening between the walls. He was fat and very dark – one of the tinkers from a camp outside the village – and he carried an armful of pots and pans.

From my vantage point I could see through the railings into the front garden where Shep was slinking noiselessly into position beneath the stones. Fascinated, I watched as the man turned unhurriedly into the opening and the dog followed the course of the disembodied head along the top of the wall.

As I expected it all happened half way along. The perfectly timed leap, the momentary pause at the summit then the tremendous 'WOOF!' into the unsuspecting ear.

It had its usual effect. I had a brief view of flailing arms and flying pans followed by a prolonged metallic clatter, then the little man reappeared like a projectile, turned right and sped away from me up the street. Considering his almost round physique he showed an astonishing turn of speed, his little legs pistoning, and he did not pause till he disappeared into the shop at the far end of the village.

I don't know why he went in there because he wouldn't find any stronger restorative than ginger pop.

Shep, apparently well satisfied, wandered back over the grass and collapsed in a cool patch where an apple tree threw its shade over the grass; head on paws he waited in comfort for his next victim.

I smiled to myself as I let in the clutch and moved off. I would stop at the shop and tell the little man that he could collect his pans without the slightest fear of being torn limb from limb, but my overriding emotion was one of relief that I had not cut the sparkle out of the big dog's life.

Shep was still having his fun.

fourteen

I suppose once you embark on a life of crime it gets easier all the time. Making a start is the only hard bit.

At any rate, that is how it seemed to me as I sat in the bus, playing hookey again. There had been absolutely no trouble about dodging out of the Grand, the streets of Scarborough had been empty of SPs and nobody had given me a second look as I strolled casually into the bus station.

It was Saturday, 13 February. Helen was expecting our baby this week-end. It could happen any time and I just didn't see how I could sit here these few miles away and do nothing. I had no classes today or tomorrow so I would miss nothing and nobody would miss me. It was, I told myself, a mere technical offence, and anyway I had no option. Like the first time, I just had to see Helen.

And it wouldn't be long now, I thought, as I hurried up to the familiar doorway of her home. I went inside and gazed disappointedly at the empty kitchen – somehow I had been sure she would be standing there waiting for me with her arms wide. I shouted her name but nothing stirred in the house. I was still there, listening, when her father came through from an inner room.

'You've got a son,' He said.

I put my hand on the back of a chair. 'What . . . ?'

'You've got a son.' He was so calm.

'When . . . ?'

'Few minutes ago. Nurse Brown's just been on the phone. Funny you should walk in.'

As I leaned on the chair he gave me a keen look. 'Would you like a drop of whisky?'

'Whisky? No – why?'

'Well you've gone a bit white, lad, that's all. Anyway, you'd better have something to eat.'

'No, no, no thanks, I've got to get out there.'

He smiled. 'There's no hurry, lad. Anyway, they won't

want anybody there too soon. Better eat something.'

'Sorry, I couldn't. Would you – would you mind if I borrowed your car?'

I was still trembling a little as I drove away. If only Mr Alderson had led up to it gradually – he might have said, 'I've got some news for you,' or something like that, but his direct approach had shattered me. When I pulled up outside Nurse Brown's it still hadn't got through to me that I was a father.

Greenside Nursing Home sounded impressive, but it was in fact Nurse Brown's dwelling house. She was State Registered and usually had two or three of the local women in at a time to have their babies.

She opened the door herself and threw up her hands. 'Mr Herriot! It hasn't taken you long! Where did you spring from?' She was a cheerfully dynamic little woman with mischievous eyes.

I smiled sheepishly. 'Well, I just happened to drop in on Mr Alderson and got the news.'

'You might have given us time to get the little fellow properly washed,' she said. 'But never mind, come up and see him. He's a fine baby – nine pounds.'

Still in a dreamlike state I followed her up the stairs of the little house into a small bedroom. Helen was there, in the bed, looking flushed.

'Hello,' she said.

I went over and kissed her.

'What was it like?' I enquired nervously.

'Awful,' Helen replied without enthusiasm. Then she nodded towards the cot beside her.

I took my first look at my son. Little Jimmy was brick red in colour and his face had a bloated, dissipated look. As I hung over him he twisted his tiny fists under his chin and appeared to be undergoing some mighty internal struggle. His face swelled and darkened as he contorted his features then from deep among the puffy flesh his eyes fixed me with a baleful glare and he stuck his tongue out of the corner of his mouth.

'My God!' I exclaimed.

The nurse looked at me, startled. 'What's the matter?'

'Well, he's a funny-looking little thing, isn't he?'

'What!' She stared at me furiously. 'Mr Herriot, how can you say such a thing? He's a beautiful baby!'

I peered into the cot again. Jimmy greeted me with a lop-sided leer, turned purple and blew a few bubbles.

'Are you sure he's all right?' I said.

There was a tired giggle from the bed but Nurse Brown was not amused.

'All right! What exactly do you mean?' She drew herself up stiffly.

I shuffled my feet. 'Well, er – is there anything wrong with him?'

I though she was going to strike me 'Anything . . . how dare you! Whatever are you talking about? I've never heard such nonsense!' She turned appealingly towards the bed, but Helen, a weary smile on her face, had closed her eyes.

I drew the enraged little woman to one side. 'Look, Nurse, have you by chance got any others on the premises?'

'Any other what?' she asked icily.

'Babies – new babies. I want to compare Jimmy with another one.'

Her eyes widened. 'Compare him! Mr Herriot, I'm not going to listen to you any longer – I've lost patience with you!'

'I'm asking you, Nurse,' I repeated. 'Have you any more around?'

There was a long pause as she looked at me as though I was something new and incredible. 'Well – there's Mrs Dewburn in the next room. Little Sidney was born about the same time as Jimmy.'

'Can I have a look at him?' I gazed at her appealingly.

She hesitated then a pitying smile crept over her face. 'Oh you . . . you . . . just a minute, then.'

She went into the other room and I heard a mumble of voices. She reappeared and beckoned to me.

Mrs Dewburn was the butcher's wife and I knew her well. The face on the pillow was hot and tired like Helen's.

'Eee, Mr Herriot, I didn't expect to see you. I thought you were in the army.'

'RAF, actually, Mrs Dewburn. I'm on – er – leave at the moment.'

I looked in the cot. Sidney was dark red and bloated, too, and he, also, seemed to be wrestling with himself. The inner battle showed in a series of grotesque facial contortions culminating in a toothless snarl.

I stepped back involuntarily. 'What a beautiful child,' I said.

'Yes, isn't he lovely,' said his mother fondly.

'He is indeed, gorgeous.' I took another disbelieving glance into the cot. 'Well, thank you very much, Mrs Dewburn. It was kind of you to let me see him.'

'Not at all, Mr Herriot, it's nice of you to take an interest.'

Outside the door I took a long breath and wiped my brow. The relief was tremendous. Sidney was even funnier than Jimmy.

When I returned to Helen's room Nurse Brown was sitting on the bed and the two women were clearly laughing at me. And of course, looking back, I must have appeared silly. Sidney Dewburn and my son are now two big, strong, remarkably good-looking young men, so my fears were groundless.

The little nurse looked at me quizzically. I think she had forgiven me.

'I suppose you think all your calves and foals are beautiful right from the moment they are born?'

'Well yes,' I replied. 'I have to admit it – I think they are.'

As I have said before, ideas do not come readily to me, but on the bus journey back to Scarborough a devilish scheme began to hatch in my brain.

I was due for compassionate leave, but why should I take it now? Helen would be in the Nursing Home for a fortnight and there didn't seem any sense in my mooning round Darrowby on my own. The thing to do would be to send myself a telegram a fortnight from now announcing the birth, and we would be able to spend my leave together.

It was interesting how my moral scruples dissolved in the face of this attraction, but anyway, I told myself, where was the harm? I wasn't scrounging anything extra, I was just altering the time. The RAF or the war effort in general would suffer no mortal blow. Long before the darkened vehicle had rolled into the town I had made up my mind and on the following day I wrote to a friend in Darrowby and arranged about the telegram.

But I wasn't such a hardened criminal as I thought, because as the days passed doubts began to creep in. The rules at ITW were rigidly strict. I would be in trouble if I was found out. But the prospect of a holiday with Helen blotted out all other considerations.

When the fateful day arrived my room mates and I were stretched on our beds after lunch when a great voice boomed along the corridor.

'AC2 Herriot! Come on, let's have you, Herriot!'

My stomach lurched. Somehow I hadn't reckoned on Flight Sergeant Blackett coming into this. I had thought maybe an LAC or a corporal, even one of the sergeants might have handled it, not the great man himself.

Flight Sergeant Blackett was an unsmiling martinet of immense natural presence which a gaunt six feet two inch frame, wide bony shoulders and a craggy countenance did nothing to diminish. It was usually the junior NCOs who dealt with our misdemeanours, but if Flight Sergeant Blackett ever took a hand it was a withering experience.

I heard it again. The same bull bellow which echoed over our heads on the square every morning.

'Herriot! Let's be having you, Herriot!'

I was on my way at a brisk trot out of the room and along the polished surface of the corridor. I came to a halt stiffly in front of the tall figure.

'Yes, Flight Sergeant.'

'You Herriot?'

'Yes, Flight Sergeant.'

The telegram between his fingers scuffed softly against the blue serge of his trousers as he swung his hand to and fro. My pulse rate accelerated painfully as I waited.

'Well now, lad, I'm pleased to tell you that your wife has had her baby safely.' He raised the telegram to his eyes. 'It says 'ere, "A boy, both well. Nurse Brown." Let me be the first to congratulate you.' He held out his hand and as I took it he smiled. Suddenly he looked very like Gary Cooper.

'Now you'll want to get off right away and see them both, eh?'

I nodded dumbly. He must have thought I was an unemotional character.

He put a hand on my shoulder and guided me into the orderly room.

'Come on, you lot, get movin'!' The organ tones rolled over the heads of the airmen seated at the tables. 'This is important. Got a brand new father 'ere. Leave pass, railway warrant, pay, double quick!'

'Right, Flight. Very good, Flight.' The typewriters began to tap.

The big man went over to a railway timetable on the wall. 'You haven't far to go, anyway. Let's see – Darrowby, Darrowby . . . yes, there's a train out of here for York at three twenty.' He looked at his watch. 'You ought to make that if you get your skates on.'

A deepening sense of shame threatened to engulf me when he spoke again.

'Double back to your room and get packed. We'll have your documents ready.'

I changed into my best blue, filled my kit bag and threw it over my shoulder, then hurried back to the orderly room.

The Flight Sergeant was waiting. He handed me a long envelope. 'It's all there, son, and you've got plenty of time.' He looked me up and down, walked round me and straightened the white flash in my cap. 'Yes, very smart. We've got to have you lookin' right for your missus, haven't we?' He gave me the Gary Cooper smile again. He was a handsome, kind-eyed man and I'd never noticed it.

He strolled with me along the corridor. 'This'll be your first 'un, of course?'

'Yes, Flight.'

He nodded. 'Well, it's a great day for you. I've got three

of 'em, meself. Getting big now but I miss 'em like hell with this ruddy war. I really envy you, walking in that door tonight and seeing your son for the very first time.'

Guilt drove through me in a searing flood and as we halted at the top of the stairs I was convinced my shifty eyes and furtive glances would betray me. But he wasn't really looking at me.

'You know, lad,' he said softly, gazing somewhere over my head. 'This is the best time of your life coming up.'

We weren't allowed to use the main stairways and as I clattered down the narrow stone service stairs I heard the big voice again.

'Give my regards to them both.'

I had a wonderful time with Helen, walking for miles, discovering the delights of pram pushing, with little Jimmy miraculously improved in appearance. Everything was so much better than if I had taken my leave at the official time and there is no doubt my plan was a success.

But I was unable to gloat about it. The triumph was dimmed and to this day I have reservations about the whole thing.

Flight Sergeant Blackett spoiled it for me.

fifteen

'You must have to be a bit of an idiot to be a country vet.' The young airman was laughing as he said it, but I felt there was some truth in his words. He had been telling me about his job in civil life and when I described my own working hours and conditions he had been incredulous.

There was one time I would have agreed with him wholeheartedly. It was nine o'clock on a filthy wet night and I was still at work. I gripped the steering wheel more tightly and shifted in my seat, groaning softly as my tired muscles complained.

Why had I entered this profession? I could have gone in for something easier and gentler – like coalmining or lumberjacking. I had started feeling sorry for myself three hours ago, driving across Darrowby market place on the way to a calving. The shops were shut and even through the wintry drizzle there was a suggestion of repose, of work done, of firesides and books and drifting tobacco smoke. I had all those things, plus Helen, back there in our bed-sitter.

I think the iron really entered when I saw the carload of young people setting off from the front of the Drovers; three girls and three young fellows, all dressed up and laughing and obviously on their way to a dance or party. Everybody was set for comfort and a good time; everybody except Herriot, rattling towards the cold wet hills and the certain prospect of toil.

And the case did nothing to raise my spirits. A skinny little heifer stretched on her side in a ramshackle openfronted shed littered with old tin cans, half bricks and other junk; it was difficult to see what I was stumbling over since the only light came from a rusty oil lamp whose flame flickered and dipped in the wind.

I was two hours in that shed, easing out the calf inch by inch. It wasn't a malpresentation, just a tight fit, but the heifer never rose to her feet and I spent the whole time on the floor, rolling among the bricks and tins, getting up only to shiver my way to the water bucket while the rain hurled itself icily against the shrinking flesh of my chest and back.

And now here I was, driving home frozen-faced with my skin chafing under my clothes and feeling as though a group of strong men had been kicking me enthusiastically from head to foot for most of the evening. I was almost drowning in self-pity when I turned into the tiny village of Copton. In the warm days of summer it was idyllic, reminding me always of a corner of Perthshire, with its single street hugging the lower slopes of a green hillside and a dark drift of trees spreading to the heathery uplands high above.

But tonight it was a dead black place with the rain sweeping across the headlights against the tight-shut houses; except for a faint glow right in the middle where the light from the village pub fell softly on the streaming roadway. I stopped the car under the swinging sign of the Fox and Hounds and on an impulse opened the door. A beer would do me good.

A pleasant warmth met me as I went into the pub. There was no bar counter, only high-backed settles and oak tables arranged under the whitewashed walls of what was simply a converted farm kitchen. At one end a wood fire crackled in an old black cooking range and above it the tick of a wall clock sounded above the murmur of voices. It wasn't as lively as the modern places but it was peaceful.

'Now then, Mr Herriot, you've been workin',' my neighbour said as I sank into the settle.

'Yes, Ted, how did you know?'

The man glanced over my soiled mackintosh and the wellingtons which I hadn't bothered to change on the farm. 'Well, that's not your Sunday suit, there's blood on your nose end and cow shit on your ear.' Ted Dobson was a burly cowman in his thirties and his white teeth showed suddenly in a wide grin.

I smiled too and plied my handkerchief. 'It's funny how you always want to scratch your nose at times like that.'

I looked around the room. There were about a dozen men drinking from pint glasses, some of them playing dominoes. They were all farm workers, the people I saw when I was called from my bed in the darkness before dawn; hunched figures they were then, shapeless in old greatcoats, cycling out to the farms, head down against the wind and rain, accepting the facts of their hard existence. I often thought at those times that this happened to me only occasionally, but they did it every morning.

And they did it for thirty shillings a week; just seeing them here made me feel a little ashamed.

Mr Waters, the landlord, whose name let him in for a certain amount of ribbing, filled my glass, holding his tall jug high to produce the professional froth.

'There y'are, Mr Herriot, that'll be sixpence. Cheap at 'alf the price.'

Every drop of beer was brought up in that jug from the wooden barrels in the cellar. It would have been totally impracticable in a busy establishment, but the Fox and Hounds was seldom bustling and Mr Waters would never get rich as a publican. But he had four cows in the little byre adjoining this room, fifty hens pecked around in his long back garden and he reared a few litters of pigs every year from his two sows.

'Thank you, Mr Waters.' I took a deep pull at the glass. I had lost some sweat despite the cold and my thirst welcomed the flow of rich nutty ale. I had been in here a few times before and the faces were all familiar. Especially old Albert Close, a retired shepherd who sat in the same place every night at the end of the settle hard against the fire.

He sat as always, his hands and chin resting on the tall crook which he had carried through his working days, his eyes blank. Stretched half under the seat, half under the table lay his dog, Mick, old and retired like his master. The animal was clearly in the middle of a vivid dream; his paws pedalled the air spasmodically, his lips and ears twitched and now and then he emitted a stifled bark.

Ted Dobson nudged me and laughed. 'Ah reckon awd Mick's still rounding up them sheep.'

I nodded. There was little doubt the dog was reliving the great days, crouching and darting, speeding in a wide arc round the perimeter of the field at his master's whistle. And Albert himself. What lay behind those empty eyes? I could imagine him in his youth, striding the windy uplands, covering endless miles over moor and rock and beck, digging that same crook into the turf at every step. There were no fitter men than the Dales shepherds, living in the open in all weathers, throwing a sack over their shoulders in snow and rain.

And there was Albert now, a broken, arthritic old man gazing apathetically from beneath the ragged peak of an ancient tweed cap. I noticed he had just drained his glass and I walked across the room.

'Good evening, Mr Close,' I said.

He cupped an ear with his hand and blinked up at me. 'Eh?'

I raised my voice to a shout. 'How are you, Mr Close?'

'Can't complain, young man,' he murmured. 'Can't complain.'

'Will you have a drink?'

'Aye, thank ye.' He directed a trembling finger at his glass. 'You can put a drop i' there, young man.'

I knew a drop meant a pint and beckoned to the landlord who plied his jug expertly. The old shepherd lifted the recharged glass and looked up at me.

'Good 'ealth,' he grunted.

'All the best,' I said and was about to return to my seat when the old dog sat up. My shouts at his master must have wakened him from his dream because he stretched sleepily, shook his head a couple of times and looked around him. And as he turned and faced me I felt a sudden sense of shock.

His eyes were terrible. In fact I could hardly see them as they winked painfully at me through a sodden fringe of pus-caked lashes. Rivulets of discharge showed dark and ugly against the white hair on either side of the nose.

I stretched my hand out to him and the dog wagged his tail briefly before closing his eyes and keeping them closed. It seemed he felt better that way.

I put my hand on Albert's shoulder. 'Mr Close, how long has he been like this?'

'Eh?'

I increased my volume. 'Mick's eyes. They're in a bad state.'

'Oh aye.' The old man nodded in comprehension. 'He's got a bit o' caud in 'em. He's allus been subjeck to it ever since 'e were a pup.'

'No, it's more than cold, it's his eyelids.'

'Eh?'

I took a deep breath and let go at the top of my voice.

'He's got turned-in eyelids. It's rather a serious thing.'

The old man nodded again. 'Aye, 'e lies a lot wi' his head at foot of t'door. It's draughty there.'

'No, Mr Close!' I bawled. 'It's got nothing to do with that. It's a thing called entropion and it needs an operation to put it right.'

'That's right, young man.' He took a sip at his beer. 'Just a bit o' caud. Ever since he were a pup he's been subjeck . . .'

I turned away wearily and returned to my seat. Ted Dobson looked at me enquiringly.

'What was that about?'

'Well, it's a nasty thing, Ted. Entropion is when the eyelids are turned in and the lashes rub against the eyeball. Causes a lot of pain, sometimes ulceration or even blindness. Even a mild case is damned uncomfortable for a dog.'

'I see,' Ted said ruminatively. 'Ah've noticed awd Mick's had mucky eyes for a long time but they've got worse lately.'

'Yes, sometimes it happens like that, but often it's congenital. I should think Mick has had a touch of it all his life but for some reason it's suddenly developed to this horrible state.' I turned again towards the old dog, sitting patiently under the table, eyes still tight shut.

'He's sufferin' then?'

I shrugged my shoulders. 'Well, you know what it's like if you have a speck of dust in your eyes or even one lash turned in. I should say he feels pretty miserable.'

'Poor awd beggar. Ah never knew it was owt like that.' He drew on his cigarette. 'And could an operation cure it?'

'Yes, Ted, it's one of the most satisfying jobs a vet can do. I always feel I've done a dog a good turn when I've finished.'

'Aye, ah bet you do. It must be a nice feelin'. But it'll be a costly job, ah reckon?'

I smiled wryly. 'It depends how you look at it. It's a fiddly business and takes time. We usually charge about a pound for it.' A human surgeon would laugh at a sum like that, but it would still be too much for old Albert.

For a few moments we were both silent, looking across the room at the old man, at the threadbare coat, the long tatter of trouser bottoms falling over the broken boots. A pound was two weeks of the old age pension. It was a fortune.

Ted got up suddenly. 'Any road, somebody ought to tell 'im. Ah'll explain it to 'im.'

He crossed the room. 'Are ye ready for another, Albert?'

The old shepherd glanced at him absently then indicated his glass, empty again. 'Aye, ye can put a drop i' there, Ted.'

The cowman waved to Mr Waters then bent down. 'Did ye understand what Mr Herriot was tellin' ye, Albert?' he shouted.

'Aye . . aye . . Mick's got a bit o' caud in 'is eyes.'

'Nay, 'e hasn't! it's nowt of t'soart! It's a en . . . a en . . . summat different.'

'Keeps gettin' caud in 'em.' Albert mumbled, nose in glass.

Ted yelled in exasperation. 'Ye daft awd divil! Listen to what ah'm sayin' – ye've got to take care of 'im and . . .'

But the old man was far away. 'Ever sin 'e were a pup . . . allus been subjeck to it . . .'

Though Mick took my mind off my own troubles at the time, the memory of those eyes haunted me for days. I yearned to get my hands on them. I knew an hour's work would transport the old dog into a world he perhaps had not known for years, and every instinct told me to rush back to Copton, throw him in the car and bear him back to Darrowby for surgery. I wasn't worried about the money but you just can't run a practice that way.

I regularly saw lame dogs on farms, skinny cats on the streets and it would have been lovely to descend on each and every one and minister to them out of my knowledge. In fact I had tried a bit of it and it didn't work.

It was Ted Dobson who put me out of my pain. He had

come in to the town to see his sister for the evening and he stood leaning on his bicycle in the surgery doorway, his cheerful, scrubbed face gleaming as if it would light up the street.

He came straight to the point. 'Will ye do that operation on awd Mick, Mr Herriot?'

'Yes, of course, but . . . how about . . . ?'

'Oh that'll be right. T'lads at Fox and Hounds are seein' to it. We're takin' it out of the club money.'

'Club money?'

'Aye, we put in a bit every week for an outin' in t'summer. Trip to t'seaside or summat like.'

'Well it's extremely kind of you, Ted, but are you quite sure? Won't any of them mind?'

Ted laughed. 'Nay, it's nowt, we won't miss a quid. We drink ower much on them do's anyway.' He paused. 'All t'lads want this job done – it's been gettin' on our bloody nerves watchin' t'awd dog ever since you told us about 'im.'

'Well, that's great,' I said. 'How will you get him down?'

'Me boss is lendin' me 'is van. Wednesday night be all right?'

'Fine.' I watched him ride away then turned back along the passage. It may seem to modern eyes that a lot of fuss had been made over a pound but in those days it was a very substantial sum, and some idea may be gained from the fact that four pounds a week was my commencing salary as a veterinary surgeon.

When Wednesday night arrived it was clear that Mick's operation had become something of a gala occasion. The little van was crammed with regulars from the Fox and Hounds and others rolled up on their bicycles.

The old dog slunk fearfully down the passage to the operating room, nostrils twitching at the unfamiliar odours of ether and antiseptic. Behind him trooped the noisy throng of farm men, their heavy boots clattering on the tiles.

Tristan, who was doing the anaesthesia, hoisted the dog on the table and I looked around at the unusual spectacle of rows of faces regarding me with keen anticipation. Normally I am not in favour of lay people witnessing operations but since these men were sponsoring the whole thing they would have to stay.

Under the lamp I got my first good look at Mick. He was a handsome, well-marked animal except for those dreadful eyes. As he sat there he opened them a fraction and peered at me for a painful moment before closing them against the bright light; that, I felt, was how he spent his life, squinting carefully and briefly at his surroundings. Giving him the intravenous barbiturate was like doing him a favour, ridding him of his torment for a while.

And when he was stretched unconscious on his side I was able to carry out my first examination. I parted the lids, wincing at the matted lashes, awash with tears and discharge; there was a long-standing keratitis and conjunctivitis but with a gush of relief I found that the cornea was not ulcerated.

'You know,' I said. 'This is a mess, but I don't think there's any permanent damage.'

The farm men didn't exactly break into a cheer but they were enormously pleased. The carnival air was heightened as they chattered and laughed and when I poised my scalpel it struck me that I had never operated in such a noisy environment.

But I felt almost gleeful as I made the first incision; I had been looking forward so much to this moment. Starting with the left eye I cut along the full length parallel to the margin of the lid then made a semicircular sweep of the knife to include half an inch of the tissue above the eye. Seizing the skin with forceps I stripped it away, and as I drew the lips of the bleeding wound together with stitches I noticed with intense gratification how the lashes were pulled high and away from the corneal surface they had irritated, perhaps for years.

I cut away less skin from the lower lid – you never need to take so much there – then started on the right eye. I was slicing away happily when I realized that the noise had subsided; there were a few mutterings, but the chaff and laughter had died. I glanced up and saw big Ken Appleton, the horseman from Laurel Grove; it was natural that he should catch my eye, because he was six feet four and built like the Shires he cared for.

'By gaw, it's 'ot in 'ere,' he whispered, and I could see he meant it because sweat was streaming down his face.

I was engrossed in my work or I would have noticed that he wasn't only sweating but deadly pale. I was stripping the skin from the eyelid when I heard Tristan's yell.

'Catch him!'

The big man's surrounding friends supported him as he slid gently to the floor and he stayed there, sleeping peacefully, till I had inserted the last stitch. Then as Tristan and I cleaned up and put the instruments away he began to look around him and his companions helped him to his feet. Now that the cutting was over the life had returned to the party and Ken came in for some leg-pulling; but his was not the only white face.

'I think you could do with a drop of whisky, Ken,' Tristan said. He left the room and returned with a bottle which, with typical hospitality, he dispensed to all. Beakers, measuring glasses and test tubes were pressed into service and soon there was a boisterous throng around the sleeping dog. When the van finally roared off into the night the last thing I heard was the sound of singing from the packed interior.

They brought Mick back in ten days for removal of the stitches. The wounds had healed well but the keratitis had still not cleared and the old dog was still blinking painfully. I didn't see the final result of my work for another month.

It was when I was again driving home through Copton from an evening call that the lighted doorway of the Fox and Hounds recalled me to the little operation which had been almost forgotten in the rush of new work. I went in and sat down among the familiar faces.

Things were uncannily like before. Old Albert Close in his usual place, Mick stretched under the table, his twitching feet testifying to another vivid dream. I watched him closely until I could stand it no longer. As if drawn by a magnet I crossed the room and crouched by him.

'Mick!' I said. 'Hey, wake up, boy!'

The quivering limbs stilled and there was a long moment when I held my breath as the shaggy head turned towards me. Then with a kind of blissful disbelief I found myself gazing into the wide, clear, bright eyes of a young dog.

Warm wine flowed richly through my veins as he faced me, mouth open in a panting grin, tail swishing along the stone flags. There was no inflammation, no discharge, and the lashes, clean and dry, grew in a soft arc well clear of the corneal surface which they had chafed and rasped for so long. I stroked his head and as he began to look around him eagerly I felt a thrill of utter delight at the sight of the old animal exulting in his freedom, savouring the new world which had opened to him. I could see Ted Dobson and the other men smiling conspiratorially as I stood up.

'Mr Close,' I shouted. 'Will you have a drink?'

'Aye, you can put a drop i' there, young man.'

'Mick's eyes are a lot better.'

The old man raised his glass. 'Good 'ealth. Aye, it were nobbut a bit o' caud.'

'But Mr Close . . . !'

'Nasty thing, is caud in t'eyes. T'awd feller keeps lyin' in that door'ole and ah reckon he'll get it again. Ever since 'e were a pup 'e's been subjeck . . .'

sixteen

As I bent over the wash basin in the 'ablutions' and went into another violent paroxysm of coughing I had a growing and uncomfortable conviction that I was a mere pawn.

The big difference between my present existence and my

old life as a vet was that I used to make up my own mind as to how I would do things, whereas in the RAF all the decisions which affected me were made by other people. I didn't much like being a pawn because the lives of us lowly airmen were ruled by a lot of notions and ideas dreamed up by individuals so exalted that we never knew them.

And so many of these ideas seemed crazy to me.

For instance, who decided that all our bedroom windows should be nailed open throughout a Yorkshire winter so that the healthy mist could swirl straight from the black ocean and settle icily on our beds as we slept? The result was an almost one hundred per cent incidence of bronchitis in our flight, and in the mornings the Grand Hotel sounded like a chest sanatorium with a harrowing chorus of barks and wheezes.

The cough seized me again, racking my body, threatening to dislodge my eyeballs. It was a temptation to report sick but I hadn't done it yet. Most of the lads stuck it out till they had roaring fevers before going sick and by now, at the end of February, nearly all of them had spent a few days in hospital. I was one of the few who hadn't. Maybe there was a bit of bravado in my stand – because most of them were eighteen- or nineteen-year-olds and I was a comparatively old man in my twenties – but there were two other reasons. Firstly, it was very often after I had got dressed and been unable to eat breakfast that I felt really ill. But by then it was too late. You had to report sick before seven o'clock or suffer till next day.

Another reason was that I didn't like the look of the sick parade. As I went out to the corridor with my towel round my shoulders a sergeant was reading a list and inflating his lungs at the same time.

'Get on parade, the sick!' he shouted. 'C'mon, c'mon, let's be 'avin' you!'

From various doors an unhappy group of invalids began to appear, shuffling over the linoleum, each draped with his 'small kit', haversack containing pyjamas, canvas shoes, knife, fork, spoon, etc.

The sergeant unleashed another bellow. 'Get into line, there! Come on, you lot, hurry it up, look lively!'

I looked at the young men huddled there, white-faced and trembling. Most of them were coughing and spluttering and one of them clutched his abdomen as though he had a ruptured appendix.

'Parade!' bawled the sergeant. 'Parade, atten-shun! Parade stan'-at ease! Atten-shun! Le-eft turn! Qui-ick march!'Eft-'ight, 'eft-'ight, 'eft-'ight, 'eft-'ight!'

The hapless band trailed wearily off. They had a march of nearly a mile through the rain to the sick quarters in another hotel above the Spa, and as I turned into my room it was with a renewed resolve to hang on as long as possible.

Another thing that frightened us all for a spell was the suggestion, drifting down from somewhere on high, that it wasn't enough to go jogging around Scarborough on our training runs; we ought to stop every now and then and do a bit of shadow boxing like fighters. This idea seemed too outrageous to be true but we had it from the sergeant himself, who came with us on our runs. Some VIP had passed it down, claiming that it would instil belligerence in us. We were thoroughly alarmed for a while, including the sergeant, who had no desire to be seen in charge of a bunch of apparent lunatics dancing around punching at the air. Mercifully, somebody had the strength to resist this one and the whole thing fell through.

But of all these brilliant schemes the one I remember best was the one that decided we had to scream at the end of our physical training session. Apart from running miles all over the place, we had long periods of PT down on the rain-swept prom with the wind cutting in from the sea on our goose-pimpled limbs. We became so good at these exercises that it was decided to put on a show for a visiting air marshal. Not only our flight but several squadrons all performing in unison in front of the Grand.

We trained for months for the big day, doing the same movements over and over again till we were perfect. At first the barrel-chested PT sergeant shouted instructions at us all the time, then as we got better all he did was call out 'Exercise three, commence.' And finally it all became so much a part of our being that he merely sounded a tiny peep on his whistle at the beginning of each exercise.

By spring we were really impressive. Hundreds of men in shorts and singlets swinging away as one out there on the square, with the PT sergeant up on the balcony above the doorway where he would stand with the air marshal on the day. The thing that made it so dramatic was the utter silence; the forest of waving limbs and swaying bodies with not a sound but the peep of the whistle.

Everything was lovely till somebody had the idea of the screaming. Up till then we had marched silently from the square at the end of the session, but that was apparently not good enough. What we had to do now was count up to five at the end of the last exercise, then leap into the air, scream at the top of our voices and run off the square at top speed.

And I had to admit that it seemed quite a brainwave. We tried it a few times, then we began to put our hearts into it, jumping high, yelling like dervishes then scuttling away into the various openings among the hotels around the square.

It must have looked marvellous from the balcony. The great mass of white-clad men going through the long routine in a cathedral hush, a few seconds of complete immobility at the end then the whole concourse erupting with a wild yell and disappearing, leaving the empty square echoing. And this last touch had another desirable aspect; it was further proof of our latent savagery. The enemy would have quaked at that chilling sound.

The sergeant had a little trouble with a lad in my flight, a tall gangling red-haired youth called Cromarty who stood in the line in front of me a few feet to my right. Cromarty seemed unable to enter into the spirit of the thing.

'Come on, lad,' the sergeant said one day. 'Put a bit of devil into it! You got to sound like a killer. You're floating up and down there like a ruddy fairy godmother.'

Cromarty did try, but the thing seemed to embarrass him. He gave a little hop, an apologetic jerk of his arms and a feeble cry.

The sergeant ran his hand through his hair. 'No, no, lad! You've got to let yourself go!' He looked around him. 'Here, Devlin, come out and show 'im how it's done.'

Devlin, a grinning Irishman, stepped forward. The scream was the high point of his day. He stood relaxed for a moment then without warning catapulted himself high in the air, legs and arms splayed, head back, while a dreadful animal cry burst from his gaping mouth.

The sergeant took an involuntary step backwards. 'Thanks, Devlin, that's fine,' he said a little shakily, then he turned to Cromarty. 'Now you see how I want it, boy, just like that. So work at it.'

Cromarty nodded. He had a long, serious face and you could see he wanted to oblige. After that I watched him each day and there was no doubt he was improving. His inhibitions were gradually being worn down.

It seemed that nature was smiling on our efforts because the great day dawned with blue skies and warm sunshine. Every man among the hundreds who marched out into the square had been individually prepared. Newly bathed, fresh haircut, spotless white shorts and singlet. We waited in our motionless lines before the newly painted door of the Grand while, on the balcony above, gold braid glinted on the air marshal's cap.

He stood among a knot of the top RAF brass of Scarborough, while in one corner I could see our sergeant, erect in long white flannels, his great chest sticking out further than ever. Beneath us the sea shimmered and the golden bay curved away to the Filey cliffs.

The sergeant raised his hand. 'Peep' went the whistle and we were off.

There was something exhilarating about being part of this smooth machine. I had a wonderful sense of oneness with the arms and legs which moved with mine all around. It was effortless. We had ten exercises to do and at the end of the first we stood rigid for ten seconds, then the whistle piped and we started again.

The time passed too quickly as I revelled in our perfection. At the end of exercise nine I came to attention, waiting for the whistle, counting under my breath. Nothing stirred, the silence was profound. Then, from the motionless ranks, as unexpected as an exploding bomb, Cromarty in front of me launched himself upwards in a tangle of flailing limbs and red hair and unleashed a long bubbling howl. He had put so much into his leap that he seemed to take a long time to come down and even after his descent the shattering sound echoed on.

Cromarty had made it at last. As fierce and warlike a scream, as high a jump as ever the sergeant could desire. The only snag was that he was too soon.

When the whistle went for the last exercise a lot of people didn't hear it because of the noise and many others were in a state of shock and came in late. Anyway, it was a shambles and the final yell and scuttle a sad anticlimax. I myself, though managing to get a few inches off the ground, was unable to make any sound at all.

Had Cromarty not been serving in the armed forces of a benign democracy he would probably have been taken quietly away and shot. As it was, there was really nothing anybody could do to him. NCOs weren't even allowed to swear at the men.

I felt for the PT sergeant. There must have been a lot he wanted to say but he was grievously restricted. I saw him with Cromarty later. He put his face close to the young man's.

'You ... you ...' His features worked as he fought for words 'You THING you!'

He turned and walked away with bowed shoulders. At that moment I'm sure he felt like a pawn too.

seventeen

may 30 1...

There is no doubt that when I looked back ... Darrowby I was inclined to bathe the whole thin... glow, but occasionally the unhappy things came to ...

That man, distraught and gasping on the surger... ...eps. 'It's no good, I can't bring him in. He's as stiff as a board!'

My stomach lurched. It was another one. 'Jasper, you mean?'

'Yes, he's in the back of my car, right here.'

I ran across the pavement and opened the car door. It was as I feared; a handsome Dalmation stretched in a dreadful tetanic spasm, spine arched, head craning desperately backward, legs like four wooden rods groping at nothing.

I didn't wait to talk but dashed back into the house for syringe and drugs.

I leaned into the car, tucked some papers under the dog's head, injected the apomorphine and waited.

The man looked at me with anxious eyes. 'What is it?'

'Strychnine poisoning, Mr Bartle. I've just given an emetic to make him vomit.' As I spoke the animal brought up the contents of his stomach on to the paper.

'Will that put him right?'

'It depends on how much of the poison has been absorbed.' I didn't feel like telling him that it was almost invariably fatal, that in fact I had treated six dogs in the last week with the same condition and they had all died. 'We'll just have to hope.'

He watched me as I filled another syringe with barbiturate. 'What are you doing now?'

'Anaesthetising him.' I slipped the needle into the radial vein and as I slowly trickled the fluid into the dog's bloodstream the taut muscles relaxed and he sank into a deep slumber.

'He looks better already,' Mr Bartle said.

'Yes, but the trouble is when the injection wears off he

...ck into a spasm. As I say, it all depends on how ... of the strychnine has got into his system. Keep him ... a quiet place with as little noise as possible. Any sound can bring on a spasm. When he shows signs of coming out of it give me a ring.'

I went back into the house. Seven cases in a week! It was tragic and scarcely believable, but there was no doubt left in my mind now. This was malicious. Some psychopath in our little town was deliberately putting down poison to kill dogs. Strychnine poisoning was something that cropped up occasionally. Gamekeepers and other people used the deadly drug to kill vermin, but usually it was handled with great care and placed out of reach of domestic pets. Trouble started when a burrowing dog came across the poison by accident. But this was different.

I had to warn pet owners somehow. I lifted the phone and spoke to one of the reporters on the *Darrowby and Houlton Times*. He promised to put the story in the next edition, along with advice to keep dogs on their leads and otherwise supervise pets more carefully.

Then I rang the police. The sergeant listened to my account. 'Right, Mr Herriot, I agree with you that there's some crackpot going around and we'll certainly investigate this matter. If you'll just give me the names of the dog owners involved ... thank you ... thank you. We'll see these people and check round the local chemists to see if anybody has been buying strychnine lately. And of course we'll keep our eyes open for anybody acting suspiciously.'

I came away from the phone feeling that I might have done something to halt the depressing series of events, but I couldn't rid myself of a gloomy apprehension that more trouble was round the corner. But my mood lightened when I saw Johnny Clifford in the waiting room.

Johnny always made me feel better because he was invariably optimistic and wore a cheerful grin which never altered, even though he was blind. He was about my own age and he sat there in his habitual pose, one hand on the head of his guide dog, Fergus.

'Is it inspection time again already, Johnny?' I asked.

'Aye, it is that, Mr Herriot, it's come round again. It's been a quick six months.' He laughed and held out his card.

I squatted and looked into the face of the big Alsatian sitting motionless and dignified by his master's side. 'Well, and how's Fergus these days?'

'Oh he's in grand fettle. Eatin' well and full of life.' The hand on the head moved round to the ears and at the other end the tail did a bit of sweeping along the waiting-room floor.

As I looked at the young man, his face alight with pride and affection, I realized afresh what this dog meant to him. He had told me that when his failing sight progressed to total blindness in his early twenties he was filled with a despair which did not lessen until he was sent to train with a guide dog and met Fergus; because he found something more than another living creature to act as his eyes, he found a friend and companion to share every moment of his days.

'Well, we'd better get started,' I said. 'Stand up a minute, old lad, while I take your temperature.' That was normal and I went over the big animal's chest with a stethoscope, listening to the reassuringly steady thud of the heart. As I parted the hair along the neck and back to examine the skin I laughed.

'I'm wasting my time here, Johnny. You've got his coat in perfect condition.'

'Aye, never a day goes by but he gets a good groomin'.'

I had seen him at it, brushing and combing tirelessly to bring extra lustre to the sleek swathes of hair. The nicest thing anybody could say to Johnny was, 'That's a beautiful dog you've got.' His pride in that beauty was boundless even though he had never seen it himself.

Treating guide dogs for the blind has always seemed to me to be one of a veterinary surgeon's most rewarding tasks. To be in a position to help and care for these magnificent animals is a privilege, not just because they are highly trained and valuable but because they represent in the ultimate way something which has always lain near the core and centre of my life: the mutually depending, trusting and loving association between man and animal.

Meeting these blind people was a humbling experience which sent me about my work with a new appreciation of my blessings.

I opened the dog's mouth and peered at the huge gleaming teeth. It was dicing with danger to do this with some Alsatians, but with Fergus you could haul the great jaws apart and nearly put your head in and he would only lick your ear. In fact he was at it now. My cheek was nicely within range and he gave it a quick wipe with his large wet tongue.

'Hey, just a minute, Fergus!' I withdrew and plied my handkerchief. 'I've had a wash this morning. And anyway, only little dogs lick – not big tough Alsatians.'

Johnny threw back his head and gave a great peal of laughter. 'There's nowt tough about him, he's the softest dog you could ever meet.'

'Well, that's the way I like them.' I said. I reached for a tooth scaler. 'There's just a bit of tartar on one of his back teeth. I'll scrape it off right now.'

When I was finished I looked in the ears with an auroscope. There was no canker but I cleaned out a little wax.

Then I went round the feet, examining paws and claws. They always fascinated me, these feet; wide, enormous, with great spreading toes. They had to be that size to support the big body and the massive bones of the limbs.

'All correct except that one funny claw, Johnny.'

'Aye, you allus have to trim that 'un don't you? I could feel it was growin' long again.'

'Yes, that toe seems to be slightly crooked or it would wear down like the others with all the walking he does. You have a great time going walks all day, don't you, Fergus?'

I dodged another attempted lick and closed my clippers around the claw. I had to squeeze till my eyes popped before the overgrown piece shot away with a loud crack.

'By gosh, we'd go through some clippers if all dogs had claws like that,' I gasped. 'It just about does them in every time he calls.'

Johnny laughed again and dropped his hand on the great head with that gesture which said so much.

I took the card and entered my report on the dog's health along with the things I had done. Then I dated it and handed it back. 'That's it for this time, Johnny. He's in excellent order and there's nothing more I need do to him.'

'Thank you, Mr Herriot. See you next time round, then.' The young man took hold of the harness and I followed the two of them along the passage and out of the front door. I watched as Fergus halted by the kerb and waited till a car had passed before crossing the road.

They hadn't gone very far along the road when a woman with a shopping bag stopped them. She began to chatter animatedly, looking down repeatedly at the big dog. She was talking about Fergus and Johnny rested his hand on the noble head and nodded and smiled. Fergus was his favourite topic.

Shortly after midday Mr Bartle rang to say Jasper showed signs of returning spasms and before sitting down to lunch I rushed round to his house and repeated the barbiturate injection. Mr Bartle owned one of the local mills, producing cattle food for the district. He was a very bright man indeed.

'Mr Herriot,' he said. 'Please don't misunderstand me. I have every faith in you, but isn't there anything else you can do? I am so very fond of this dog.'

I shrugged helplessly. 'I'm sorry, but I can't do any more.'

'But is there no antidote to this poison?'

'No, I'm afraid there isn't.'

'Well ...' He looked down with drawn face at the unconscious animal. 'What's going on? What's happening to Jasper when he goes stiff like he did? I'm only a layman but I like to understand things.'

'I'll try to explain it,' I said. 'Strychnine is absorbed into the nervous system and it increases the conductivity of the spinal cord.'

'What does that mean?'

'It means that the muscles become more sensitive to outside stimuli so that the slightest touch or sound throws them into violent contractions.'

'But why does a dog stretch out like that?'

'Because the extensor muscles are stronger than the flexors, causing the back to be arched and the legs extended.'

He nodded. 'I see, but . . . I believe it is usually fatal. What is it that . . . that kills them?'

'They die of asphyxia due to paralysis of the respiratory centre or contraction of the diaphragm.'

Maybe he wanted to ask more, but it was painful for him and he stayed silent.

'There's one thing I'd like you to know, Mr Bartle,' I said. 'It is almost certainly not a painful condition.'

'Thank you.' He bent and briefly stroked the sleeping dog. 'So nothing more can be done?'

I shook my head. 'The barbiturate keeps the spasms in abeyance and we'll go on hoping he hasn't absorbed too much strychnine. I'll call back later, or you can ring me if he gets worse. I can be here in a few minutes.'

Driving away, I pondered on the irony that made Darrowby a paradise for dog killers as well as dog lovers. There were grassy tracks everywhere; wandering by the river's edge, climbing the fell-sides and coiling green and tempting among the heather on the high tops. I often felt sympathy for pet owners in the big cities, trying to find places to walk their dogs. Here in Darrowby we could take our pick. But so could the poisoner. He could drop his deadly bait unobserved in a hundred different places.

I was finishing the afternoon surgery when the phone rang. It was Mr Bartle.

'Has he started the spasms again?' I asked.

There was a pause. 'No, I'm afraid Jasper is dead. He never regained consciousness.'

'Oh . . . I'm very sorry.' I felt a dull despair. That was the seventh death in a week.

'Well, thank you for your treatment, Mr Herriot. I'm sure nothing could have saved him.'

I hung up the phone wearily. He was right. Nothing or nobody could have done any good in this case, but it didn't help. If you finish up with a dead animal there is always the feeling of defeat.

Next day I was walking on to a farm when the farmer's wife called to me. 'I have a message for you to ring back to the surgery.'

I heard Helen's voice at the other end. 'Jack Brimham has just come in with his dog. I think it's another strychnine case.'

I excused myself and drove back to Darrowby at top speed. Jack Brimham was a builder. He ran a one-man business and whatever job he was on – repairing roofs or walls or chimneys – his little white rough-haired terrier went with him, and you could usually see the little animal nosing among the piles of bricks, exploring in the surrounding fields.

Jack was a friend, too. I often had a beer with him at the Drovers' Arms and I recognized his van outside the surgery. I trotted along the passage and found him leaning over the table in the consulting room. His dog was stretched there in that attitude which I dreaded.

'He's gone, Jim,' he muttered.

I looked at the shaggy little body. There was no movement, the eyes stared silently. The legs, even in death strained across the smooth surface of the table. It was pointless, but I slipped my hand inside the thigh and felt for the femoral artery. There was no pulse.

'I'm sorry, Jack,' I said.

He didn't answer for a moment. 'I've been readin' about this in the paper, Jim, but I never thought it would happen to me. It's a bugger, isn't it?'

I nodded. He was a craggy-faced man, a tough Yorkshireman with a humour and integrity which I liked and a soft place inside which his dog had occupied. I did not know what to say to him.

'Who's doin' this?' he said, half to himself.

'I don't know, Jack. Nobody knows.'

'Well I wish I could have five minutes with him, that's all.' He gathered the rigid little form into his arms and went out.

My troubles were not over for that day. It was about 11 p.m. and I had just got into bed when Helen nudged me.

'I think there's somebody knocking at the front door, Jim.'

I opened the window and looked out. Old Boardman, the lame veteran of the first war who did odd jobs for us, was standing on the steps.

'Mr Herriot,' he called up to me. 'I'm sorry to bother you at this hour, but Patch is ill.'

I leaned further out. 'What's he doing?'

'He's like a bit o' wood – stiff like, and laid on 'is side.'

I didn't bother to dress, just pulled my working corduroys over my pyjamas and went down the stairs two at a time. I grabbed what I needed from the dispensary and opened the front door. The old man, in shirt sleeves, caught at my arm.

'Come quickly, Mr Herriot!' He limped ahead of me to his little house about twenty yards away in the lane round the corner.

Patch was like all the others. The fat spaniel I had seen so often waddling round the top yard with his master was in that nightmare position on the kitchen floor, but he had vomited, which gave me hope. I administered the intravenous injection but as I withdrew the needle the breathing stopped.

Mrs Boardman, in nightgown and slippers, dropped on her knees and stretched a trembling hand towards the motionless animal.

'Patch . . .' She turned and stared at me, wide-eyed. 'He's dead!'

I put my hand on the old woman's shoulder and said some sympathetic words. I thought grimly that I was getting good at it. As I left I looked back at the two old people. Boardman was kneeling now by his wife and even after I had closed the door I could hear their voices: 'Patch . . . oh Patch.'

I almost reeled over the few steps to Skeldale House and before going in I stood in the empty street breathing the cool air and trying to calm my racing thoughts. With Patch gone, the thing was getting very near home. I saw that dog every day. In fact all the dogs that had died were old friends – in a little town like Darrowby you came to know your patients personally. Where was it going to end?

I didn't sleep much that night and over the next few days I was obsessed with apprehension. I expected another poisoning with every phone call and took care never to let my own dog, Sam, out of the car in the region of the town. Thanks to my job I was able to exercise him miles away on the summits of the fells, but even there I kept him close to me.

By the fourth day I was beginning to feel more relaxed. Maybe the nightmare was over. I was driving home in the late afternoon past the row of grey cottages at the end of the Houlton Road when a woman ran waving into the road.

'Oh, Mr Herriot,' she cried when I stopped. 'I was just goin' to t'phone box when I saw you.'

I pulled up by the kerb. 'It's Mrs Clifford, isn't it?'

'Yes, Johnny's just come in and Fergus 'as gone queer. Collapsed and laid on t'floor.'

'Oh no!' An icy chill drove through me and for a moment I stared at her, unable to move. Then I threw open the car door and hurried after Johnny's mother into the end cottage. I halted abruptly in the little room and stared down in horror. The very sight of the splendid dignified animal scrabbling helplessly on the linoleum was a desecration, but strychnine is no respecter of such things.

'Oh God!' I breathed. 'Has he vomited, Johnny?'

'Aye, me mum said he was sick in t'back garden when we came in.' The young man was sitting very upright in a chair by the side of his dog. Even now there was a half smile on his face, but he looked strained as he put out his hand in the old gesture and failed to find the head that should have been there.

The bottle of barbiturate wobbled in my shaking hand as I filled the syringe. I tried to put away the thought that I was doing what I had done to all the others – all the dead ones. At my feet Fergus panted desperately, then as I bent over him he suddenly became still and went into the horrible distinctive spasm, the great limbs I knew so well straining frantically into space, the head pulled back grotesquely over the spine.

This was when they died, when the muscles were at full contraction. As the barbiturate flowed into the vein I waited for signs of relaxation but saw none. Fergus was about twice as heavy as any of the other victims I had treated and the plunger went to the end of the syringe without result.

Quickly I drew in another dose and began to inject it, my tension building as I saw how much I was administering. The recommended dose was 1 cc per 5 lb body weight and beyond that you could kill the animal. I watched the gradations on the glass barrel of the syringe and my mouth went dry when the dose crept far beyond the safety limit. But I knew I had to relieve this spasm and continued to depress the plunger relentlessly.

I did it in the grim knowledge that if he died now I would never know whether to blame the strychnine or myself for his death.

The big dog had received more than a lethal amount before peace began to return to the taut body and even then I sat back on my heels, almost afraid to look in case I had brought about his end. There was a long agonizing moment when he lay still and apparently lifeless then the rib cage began to move almost imperceptibly as the breathing recommenced.

Even then I was in suspense. The anaesthesia was so deep that he was only just alive, yet I knew that the only hope was to keep him that way. I sent Mrs Clifford out to phone Siegfried that I would be tied up here for a while, then I pulled up a chair and settled down to wait.

The hours passed as Johnny and I sat there, the dog stretched between us. The young man discussed the case calmly and without self-pity. There was no suggestion that this was anything more than a pet animal lying at his feet – except for the tell-tale reaching for the head that was no longer there.

Several times Fergus showed signs of going into another spasm and each time I sent him back into his deep, deep insensibility, pushing him repeatedly to the brink with a fateful certainty that it was the only way.

It was well after midnight when I came sleepily out into the darkness. I felt drained. Watching the life of the friendly, clever, face-licking animal flicker as he lay inert and unheeding had been a tremendous strain, but I had left him sleeping – still anaesthetized but breathing deeply and regularly. Would he wake up and start the dread sequence again? I didn't know and I couldn't stay any longer. There was a practice with other animals to attend to.

But my anxiety jerked me into early wakefulness next morning. I tossed around till seven thirty telling myself this wasn't the way to be a veterinary surgeon, that you couldn't live like this. But my worry was stronger than the voice of reason and I slipped out before breakfast to the roadside cottage.

My nerves were like a bowstring as I knocked on the door. Mrs Clifford answered and I was about to blurt out my enquiries when Fergus trotted from the inner room.

He was still a little groggy from the vast dosage of barbiturate but he was relaxed and happy, the symptoms had gone, he was himself again. With a gush of pure joy I knelt and took the great head between my hands. He slobbered at me playfully with his wet tongue and I had to fight him off.

He followed me into the living room where Johnny was seated at the table, drinking tea. He took up his usual position, sitting upright and proud by his master's side.

'You'll have a cup, Mr Herriot?' Mrs Clifford asked, poising the teapot.

'Thanks, I'd love one, Mrs Clifford,' I replied.

No tea ever tasted better and as I sipped I watched the young man's smiling face.

'What a relief, Mr Herriot! I sat up with him all night, listenin' to the chimes of the church clock. It was just after four when I knew we'd won because I heard 'im get to his feet and sort o' stagger about. I stopped worryin' then, just listened to 'is feet patterin' on the linoleum. It was lovely!'

He turned his head to me and I looked at the slightly up-turned eyes in the cheerful face.

'I'd have been lost without Fergus,' he said softly. 'I don't know how to thank you.'

But as he unthinkingly rested his hand on the head of the big dog who was his pride and delight I felt that the gesture alone was all the thanks I wanted.

That was the end of the strychnine poisoning outbreak in Darrowby. The older people still talk about it, but nobody ever had the slightest clue to the identity of the killer and it is a mystery to this day.

I feel that the vigilance of the police and the publicity in the press frightened this twisted person off, but anyway it just stopped and the only cases since then have been accidental ones.

To me it is a sad memory of failure and frustration. Fergus was my only cure and I'm not sure why he recovered. Maybe the fact that I pushed the injection to dangerous levels because I was desperate had something to do with it, or maybe he just didn't pick up as much poison as the others. I'll never know.

But over the years when I saw the big dog striding majestically in his harness, leading his master unerringly around the streets of Darrowby, I always had the same feeling.

If there had to be just one saved, I'm glad it was him.

eighteen

A tender nerve twinged as the old lady passed me the cup of tea. She looked just like Mrs Beck.

One of the local churches was having a social evening to entertain us lonely airmen and as I accepted the cup and sat down I could hardly withdraw my eyes from the lady's face.

Mrs Beck! I could see her now standing by the surgery window.

'Oooh, I never thought you were such a 'eartless man, Mr Herriot.' Her chin trembled and she looked up at me reproachfully.

'But Mrs Beck,' I said. 'I assure you I am not being in the least heartless. I just cannot carry out a major operation on your cat for ten shillings.'

'Well, I thought you would've done it for a poor widder woman like me.'

I regarded her thoughtfully, taking in the small compact figure, the healthy cheeks, the neat helmet of grey hair pulled tightly into a bun. Was she really a poor widow? There was cause for doubt. Her next-door neighbour in Rayton village was a confirmed sceptic.

'It's all a tale, Mr Herriot,' he had said. 'She tries it on wi' everybody, but I'll tell you this – she's got a long stockin'. Owns property all over t'place.'

I took a deep breath. 'Mrs Beck. We often do work at reduced rates for people who can't afford to pay, but this is what we call a luxury operation.'

'Luxury!' The lady was aghast. 'Eee, ah've been tellin' you how Georgina keeps havin' them kittens. She's at it all the time and it's gettin' me down. Ah can't sleep for worryin' when t'next lot's comin'.' She dabbed her eyes.

'I understand and I'm sorry. I can only tell you again that the only way to prevent this trouble is to spay your cat and the charge is one pound.'

'Nay, I can't afford that much!'

I spread my hands. 'But you are asking me to do it for half the price. That's ridiculous. This operation involves the removal of the uterus and ovaries under a general anaesthetic. You just can't do a job like that for ten shillings.'

'Oh, you are cruel!' She turned and looked out of the window and her shoulders began to shake. 'You won't even take pity on a poor widder.'

This had been going on for ten minutes and it began to dawn on me that I was in the presence of a stronger character than myself. I glanced at my watch – I should have been on my round by now and it was becoming increasingly obvious that I wasn't going to win this argument.

I sighed. Maybe she really was a poor widow. 'All right, Mrs Beck, I'll do it for ten shillings, just this once. Will Tuesday afternoon be all right for you?'

She swung round from the window, her face crinkling magically into a smile. 'That'll suit me grand! Eee, that's right kind of you.' She tripped past me and I followed her along the passage.

'Just one thing,' I said as I held the front door open for her. 'Don't give Georgina any food from midday on Monday. She must have an empty stomach when you bring her in.'

'Bring 'er in?' She was a picture of bewilderment. 'But I 'aven't got no car. I thought you'd be collectin' her.'

'Collecting! But Rayton's five miles away!'

'Yes, and bring 'er back afterwards, too. I 'ave no transport.'

'Collect . . . operate on her . . . take her back! All for ten shillings!'

She was still smiling but a touch of steel glinted in her eyes. 'Well, that's what you agreed to charge – ten shillings.'

'But . . . but . . .'

'Oh now you're startin' again.' The smile faded and she put her head on one side. 'And I'm only a poor . . .'

'Okay, okay,' I said hastily. 'I'll call on Tuesday.'

And when Tuesday afternoon came round I cursed my

softness. If that cat had been brought in I could have operated on her at two o'clock and been out on the road doing my farm calls by two thirty. I didn't mind working at a loss for half an hour, but how long was this business going to take?

On my way out I glanced through the open door of the sitting room. Tristan was supposed to be studying but was sleeping soundly in his favourite chair. I went in and looked down at him, marvelling at the utter relaxation, seen only in a dedicated sleeper. His face was as smooth and untroubled as a baby's, the *Daily Mirror*, open at the comic strips, had fallen across his chest and a burnt-out Woodbine hung from one dangling hand.

I shook him gently. 'Like to come with me, Triss? I've got to pick up a cat.'

He came round slowly, stretching and grimacing, but his fundamental good nature soon reasserted itself.

'Certainly, Jim,' he said with a final yawn. 'It will be a pleasure.'

Mrs Beck lived half way down the left side of Rayton village. I read 'Jasmine Cottage' on the brightly painted gate, and as we went up the garden path the door opened and the little woman waved gaily.

'Good afternoon, gentlemen, I'm right glad to see you both.' She ushered us into the living-room among good, solid-looking furniture which showed no sign of poverty. The open cupboard of a mahogany sideboard gave me a glimpse of glasses and bottles. I managed to identify Scotch, cherry brandy and sherry before she nudged the door shut with her knee.

I pointed to a cardboard box loosely tied with string. 'Ah, good, you've got her in there, have you?'

'Nay, bless you, she's in t'garden. She allus has a bit of play out there of an afternoon.'

'In the garden, eh?' I said nervously. 'Well, please get her in, we're in rather a hurry.'

We went through a tiled kitchen to the back door. Most of these cottages had a surprising amount of land behind them and Mrs Beck's patch was in very nice order. Flower beds bordered a smooth stretch of lawn and the sunshine drew glittering colours from the apples and pears among the branches of the trees.

'Georgina,' carolled Mrs Beck. 'Where are you, my pet?'

No cat appeared and she turned to me with a roguish smile. 'I think the little imp's playin' a game with us. She does that, you know.'

'Really?' I said without enthusiasm. 'Well, I wish she'd show herself. I really don't have much . . .'

At that moment a very fat tabby darted from a patch of chrysanthemums and flitted across the grass into a clump of rhododendrons with Tristan in close pursuit. The young man dived among the greenery and the cat emerged from the other end at top speed, did a couple of laps of the lawn then shot up a gnarled tree.

Tristan, eyes gleaming in anticipation, lifted a couple of windfall apples from the turf. 'I'll soon shift the bugger from there, Jim,' he whispered and took aim.

I grabbed his arm. 'For heaven's sake, Triss!' I hissed. 'You can't do that. Put those things down.'

'Oh . . . all right.' He dropped the apples and made for the tree. 'I'll get hold of her for you, anyway.'

'Wait a minute.' I seized his coat as he passed. 'I'll do it. You stay down here and try to catch her if she jumps.'

Tristan looked disappointed but I gave him a warning look. The way the cat had moved, it struck me that it only needed a bit of my colleague's ebullience to send the animal winging into the next county. I began to climb the tree.

I like cats, I've always liked them, and since I feel that animals recognize this in a person I have usually been able to approach and handle the most difficult types. It is not too much to say that I prided myself on my cat technique; I didn't foresee any trouble here.

Puffing slightly, I reached the top branch and extended a hand to the crouching animal.

'Pooss-pooss,' I cooed, using my irresistible cat tone.

Georgina eyed me coldly and gave no answering sign other than a higher arching of the back.

I leaned further along the branch. 'Pooss-pooss, pooss-pooss.' My voice was like molten honey, my finger near her face. I would rub her cheek ever so gently and she would be mine. It never failed.

'Pah!' replied Georgina warningly but I took no heed and touched the fur under her chin.

'Pah-pah!' Georgina spat and followed with a lightning left hook which opened a bloody track across the back of my hand.

Muttering fervently, I retreated and nursed my wounds. From below Mrs Beck gave a tinkling laugh.

'Oh, isn't she a little monkey! She's that playful, bless her.'

I snorted and began to ease my way along the branch again. This time, I thought grimly, I would dispense with finesse. The quick grab was indicated here.

As though reading my thoughts the little creature tripped to the end of the branch and as it bent low under her weight she dropped lightly to the grass.

Tristan was on her in a flash, throwing himself full length and seizing her by the hind leg. Georgina whipped round and unhesitatingly sank her teeth into his thumb but Tristan's core of resilience showed. After a single howl of agony he changed his grip at lightning speed to the scruff of the neck.

A moment later he was standing upright holding a dangling fighting fury high in the air.

'Right, Jim,' he called happily. 'I have her.'

'Good lad! Hang on!' I said breathlessly and slithered down the tree as quickly as I could. Too quickly, in fact, as an ominous ripping sound announced the removal of a triangular piece of my jacket elbow.

But I couldn't bother with trifles. Ushering Tristan at a gallop into the house I opened the cardboard box. There were no sophisticated cat containers in those days and it was a tricky job to enclose Georgina, who was lashing out in all directions and complaining bitterly in a bad-tempered wail.

It took a panting ten minutes to imprison the cat but even with several yards of rough twine round the floppy cardboard I still didn't feel very secure as I bore it to the car.

Mrs Beck raised a finger as we were about to drive away. I carefully explored my lacerated hand and Tristan sucked his thumb as we waited for her to speak.

'Mr Herriot, I 'ope you'll be gentle with 'er,' she said anxiously. 'She's very timid, you know.'

We had covered barely half a mile before sounds of strife arose from the back.

'Get back! Get in there. Get back, you bugger!'

I glanced behind me. Tristan was having trouble. Georgina clearly didn't care for the motion of the car and from the slits in the box clawed feet issued repeatedly; on one occasion an enraged spitting face got free as far as the neck. Tristan kept pushing everything back with great resolution but I could tell from the rising desperation of his cries that he was fighting a losing battle.

I heard the final shout with a feeling of inevitability.

'She's out, Jim! The bugger's out!'

Well this was great. Anybody who has driven a car with a hysterical cat hurtling around the interior will appreciate my situation. I crouched low over the wheel as the furry creature streaked round the sides or leaped clawing at the roof or windscreen with Tristan lunging vainly after her.

But cruel fate had not finished with us yet. My colleague's gaps and grunts from the rear ceased for a moment to be replaced by a horrified shriek.

'The bloody thing's shitting, Jim! She's shitting everywhere!'

The cat was obviously using every weapon at her disposal and he didn't have to tell me. My nose was way ahead of him, and I frantically wound down the window. But I closed it just as quickly at the rising image of Georgina escaping and disappearing into the unknown.

I don't like to think of the rest of that journey. I tried to breathe through my mouth and Tristan puffed out dense clouds of Woodbine smoke but it was still pretty terrible.

Just outside Darrowby I stopped the car and we made a concerted onslaught on the animal; at the cost of a few more wounds, including a particularly painful scratch on my nose, we cornered her and fastened her once more in the box.

Even on the operating table Georgina had a few tricks left. We were using ether and oxygen as anaesthetic and she was particularly adept at holding her breath while the mask was on her face then returning suddenly to violent life when we thought she was asleep. We were both sweating when she finally went under.

I suppose it was inevitable, too, that she should be a difficult case. Ovaro-hysterectomy in the cat is a fairly straightforward procedure and nowadays we do innumerable cases uneventfully, but in the thirties, particularly in country practice, it was infrequently done and consequently a much larger undertaking.

I personally had my own preferences and aversions in this field. For instance, I found thin cats easy to do and fat cats difficult. Georgina was extremely fat.

When I opened her abdomen an ocean of fat welled up at me, obscuring everything, and I spent a long nerve-racking period lifting out portions of bowel or omentum with my forceps, surveying them gloomily and stuffing them back in again. A great weariness had begun to creep over me by the time I at last managed to grip the pink ovary between the metallic jaws and drew forth the slender string of uterus. After that it was routine, but I still felt a strange sense of exhaustion as I inserted the last stitch.

I put the sleeping cat into the box and beckoned to Tristan. 'Come on, let's get her home before she comes round.' I was starting along the passage when he put his hand on my arm.

'Jim,' he said gravely. 'You know I'm your friend.'

'Yes, Triss, of course.'

'I'd do anything for you, Jim.'

'I'm sure you would.'

He took a deep breath. 'Except one thing. I'm not going back in that bloody car.'

I nodded dully. I really couldn't blame him.

'That's all right,' I said. 'I'll be off, then.'

Before leaving I sprinkled the interior with pine-smelling disinfectant but it didn't make much difference. In any case my main emotion was the hope that Georgina wouldn't wake up before I got to Rayton, and that was shattered before I had crossed Darrowby market place. The hair prickled on the back of my neck as an ominous droning issued from the box on the rear seat. It was like the sound of a distant swarm of bees but I knew what it meant; the anaesthetic was wearing off.

Once clear of the town I put my foot on the boards. This was something I rarely did because whenever I pushed my vehicle above forty miles an hour there was such a clamour of protest from engine and body that I always feared the thing would disintegrate around me. But at this moment I didn't care. Teeth clenched, eyes staring, I hurtled forward, but I didn't see the lonely strip of tarmac or the stone walls flitting past; all my attention was focused behind me, where the swarm of bees was getting nearer and the tone angrier.

When it developed into a bad-tempered yowling and was accompanied by the sound of strong claws tearing at cardboard I began to tremble. As I thundered into Rayton village I glanced behind me. Georgina was half out of the box. I reached back and grasped her scruff and when I stopped at the gate of Jasmine Cottage I pulled on the brake with one hand and lifted her on to my lap with the other.

I sagged in the seat, my breath escaping in a great explosion of relief; and my stiff features almost bent into a smile as I saw Mrs Beck pottering in her garden.

She took Georgina from me with a cry of joy but gasped in horror when she saw the shaven area and the two stitches on the cat's flank.

'Oooh, my darlin'! What 'ave those nasty men been doin' to you?' She hugged the animal to her and glared at me.

'She's all right, Mrs Beck, she's fine,' I said. 'You can give her a little milk tonight and some solid food tomorrow. There's nothing to worry about.'

She pouted. 'Oh, very well. And now . . .' She gave me a sidelong glance. 'I suppose you'll want your money?'

'Well, er . . .'

'Wait there, then. I'll get it.' She turned and went into the house.

Standing there, leaning against the reeking car, feeling the sting of the scratches on my hands and nose and examining the long tear on my jacket elbow I felt physically and emotionally spent. All I had done this afternoon was spay a cat but I had nothing more to offer.

Apathetically I watched the lady coming down the path. She was carrying a purse. At the gate she stopped and faced me.

'Ten shillin's, wasn't it?'

'That's right.'

She rummaged in the purse for some time before pulling out a ten-shilling note which was regarded sadly.

'Oh Georgina, Georgina, you *are* an expensive pussy,' she soliloquized.

Tentatively I began to extend my hand but she pulled the note away. 'Just a minute, I'm forgettin'. You 'ave to take the stitches out, don't you?'

'Yes, in ten days.'

She set her lips firmly. 'Well there's plenty of time to pay ye then – ye'll be here again.'

'Here again . . . ? But you can't expect . . .'

'I allus think it's unlucky to pay afore a job's finished,' she said. 'Summat terrible might happen to Georgina.'

'But . . . but . . .'

'Nay, ah've made up me mind,' she said. She replaced the money and snapped the purse shut with an air of finality before turning towards the house. Halfway up the path she looked over her shoulder and smiled.

'Aye, that's what I'll do. I'll pay ye when ye come back.'

nineteen

We were ready to march away from Scarborough. And it was ironical that we were leaving just when the place was beginning to smile on us.

In the May sunshine we stood on parade outside the Grand at 7 a.m. as we had done throughout the Yorkshire winter, mostly in darkness, often with the icy rain blowing in our faces. But now I felt a pang of regret as I looked over the heads at the wide beautiful bay stretching beneath its cliffs to the far headland, the sand clean-washed and inviting, the great blue expanse of sea shimmering and glittering and over everything the delicious sea-smell of salt and seaweed, raising memories of holidays and happy things lost in the war.

'Atten-shun!' Flight Sergeant Blackett's bellow rolled over us as we stiffened in our ranks, every man carrying full kit, our packs braced with sheets of cardboard to give the sharp, rectangular look, hair cut short, boots gleaming, buttons shining like gold. Without our knowing, No. ten ITW had moulded us into a smart, disciplined unit, very different from the shambling, half-baked crew of six months ago. We had all passed our exams and were no longer AC2s but Leading Aircraftmen, and as LAC Herriot my wage had rocketed from three shillings to a dizzying seven and three-pence a day.

'Right turn!' Again the roar. 'By the left qui-ick march!'

Arms high, moving as one, we swung past the front of the Grand for the last time. I shot a parting glance at the great building – like a dignified Victorian lady stripped of her finery – and I made a resolve. I would come back some day, when the war was over, and see the Grand Hotel as it should be.

And I did, too. Years later, Helen and I sat in deep arm-chairs in the lounge where the SPs had barked. Waiters padded over the thick carpets with tea and muffins while a string orchestra played selections from *Rose Marie*.

And in the evening we dined in the elegant room with its long unbroken line of window looking down on the sea. This room had been the cold open terrace where I learned to read the Aldis lamp flickering from the lighthouse, but now we sat in luxurious warmth eating grilled sole and watching the lights of the harbour and town beginning to wink in the gathering dusk.

But that was very much in the future as the tramping feet echoed along Huntriss Row on the way to the station and the long lines of blue left the emptying square. We didn't know where we were going, everything was uncertain.

Black's *Veterinary Dictionary* dug into my back through the layer of cardboard. It was an unwieldy article but it reminded me of good days and gave me hope of more to come.

twenty

'It's the same the whole world over, it's the poor wot gets the blame. It's the rich wot gets the pleasure . . .'

We were on a 'toughening course', living under canvas in the depths of Shropshire, and this was one of the occasions when we were all gathered together – hundreds of sunburned men – in a huge marquee waiting to be addressed by a visiting air commodore.

Before the great man arrived the platform was occupied by a lascivious sergeant who was whittling away the time by leading us in a succession of bawdy ditties accompanied by gestures. 'It's the rich wot gets the . . .', but instead of 'pleasure' he made a series of violent pumping movements with his forearm.

I was intrigued by the reaction of the airman on my right. He was a slim, pink-faced lad of about nineteen and his lank fair hair fell over his face as he jumped up and down. He was really throwing himself into it, bawling out the indelicate words, duplicating the sergeant's gesticulations with maniacal glee. He was, I had recently learned, the son of a bishop.

We had been joined on this course by the Oxford University Air Squadron. They were a group of superior and delicately nurtured young men and since I had spent three full days peeling potatoes with them I had come to know most of them very well. 'Spud bashing' is an unequalled method of becoming familiar with one's fellow men and as, hour after hour, we filled countless bins with our produce, the barriers crumbled steadily until at the end of three days we didn't have many secrets from each other.

The bishop's son had found something hilarious in the idea of a qualified veterinary surgeon leaving his practice to succour his country by removing the skins from thousands of tubers. And I, on the other hand, derived some reward from watching his antics. He was a charming and likeable lad but he seized avidly on anything with the faintest salacious slant. They say parsons' sons are a bit wild when let off the leash, and I suppose an escapee from a bishop's palace is even more susceptible to the blandishments of the big world.

I looked at him again. All around him men were yelling their heads off, but his voice, mouthing the four-letter words with relish, rang above the rest and he followed the actions of the conducting sergeant like a devoted acolyte.

It was all so different from Darrowby. My early days in the RAF with all the swearing and uninhibited conversation made me realize, perhaps for the first time, what kind of a community I had left behind me. Because I often think that one of the least permissive societies in the history of mankind was the agricultural community of rural Yorkshire in the thirties. Among the farmers anything to do with sex or the natural functions was unmentionable.

It made my work more difficult because if the animal's ailment had the slightest sexual connotation its owner would refuse to go into details if Helen or our secretary Miss

Harbottle answered the phone. 'I want the vet to come and see a cow,' was as far as they would go.

Today's case was typical and I looked at Mr Hopps with some irritation.

'Why didn't you say your cow wasn't coming into season? There's a new injection for that now but I haven't got it with me. I can't carry everything in my car, you know.'

The farmer studied his feet. 'Well, it was a lady on t'phone and I didn't like to tell 'er that Snowdrop wasn't bullin'.' He looked up at me sheepishly. 'Can't you do owt about it, then?'

I sighed. 'Maybe I can. Bring me a bucket of hot water and some soap.'

As I lathered my arm I felt a twinge of disappointment. I'd have liked to try that new Prolan injection. But on the other hand there was a certain interest in these rectal examinations.

'Hold her tail, please,' I said, and began to work my hand carefully past the anal ring.

We were doing a lot of this lately. The profession had awakened quite suddenly to the fact that bovine infertility was no longer an impenetrable mystery. We were carrying out more and more of these examinations, and as I say, they had a strange fascination.

Siegfried put it with his usual succinctness one morning.

'James,' he said. 'There is more to be learned up a cow's arse than in many an encyclopaedia.'

And, groping my way into this animal, I could see what he meant. Through the rectal wall I gripped the uterine cervix, then I worked along the right horn. It felt perfectly normal, as did the fallopian tube when I reached it. In another moment the ovary rested between my fingers like a walnut; but it was a walnut with a significant bulge and I smiled to myself. That swelling was the corpus luteum, the 'yellow body' which was exerting its influence on the ovary and preventing the initiation of the normal oestral cycle.

I squeezed gently on the base of the bulge and felt it part from the ovary and swim off into space. That was lovely – just what was required – and I looked happily along the cow's back at the farmer.

'I think I've put things right, Mr Hopps. She should come on within the next day or two and you can get her served right away.'

I withdrew my arm, smeared with filth almost to the shoulder, and began to swill it with the warm water. This was the moment when young people with dewy-eyed ambitions to be veterinary surgeons usually decided to be lawyers or nurses instead. A lot of teenagers came round with me to see practice and it seemed to me that the sooner they witnessed the realities of the job the better it would be for them. A morning's pregnancy diagnoses or something similar had a salutary effect in sorting out the sheep from the goats.

As I left the farm I had the satisfied feeling that I had really done something, and a sensation of relief that Mr Hopps' delicacy hadn't resulted in an abortive visit.

It was strange, but when I returned to the surgery I immediately encountered another example of the same thing.

Mr Pinkerton, a smallholder, was sitting in the office next to Miss Harbottle's desk. By his side sat his farm collie.

'Well, what can I do for you, Mr Pinkerton?' I asked as I closed the door behind me.

The farmer hesitated. 'It's me dog – 'e isn't right.'

'What do you mean? Is he ill?' I bent down and stroked the shaggy head and as the dog leaped up in delight his tail began to beat a booming tom-tom rhythm against the side of the desk.

'Nay, nay, he's right enough in 'imself.' The man was clearly ill at ease.

'Well, what's the trouble? He looks the picture of health to me.'

'Aye, but ah'm a bit worried. Ye see it's 'is . . .' He glanced furtively towards Miss Harbottle. 'It's 'is pencil.'

'What d'you say?'

A faint flush mounted in Mr Pinkerton's thin cheeks. Again he shot a terrified glance at Miss Harbottle. 'It's 'is . . . pencil. There's summat matter with 'is pencil.' He indicated by the merest twitch of his forefinger somewhere in the direction of the animal's belly.

I looked. 'I'm sorry, but I can't see anything unusual.'

'Ah, but there is.' The farmer's face twisted in an agony of embarrassment and he pushed his face close to mine. 'There's summat there,' he said in a hoarse whisper. 'Summat comin' from 'is . . . 'is pencil.'

I got down on my knees and had a closer look, and suddenly all became clear.

'Is that what you mean?' I pointed to a tiny blob of semen on the end of the prepuce.

He nodded dumbly, his face a study in woe.

I laughed. 'Well you can stop worrying. That's nothing abnormal. You might call it an overflow. He's just a young dog, isn't he?'

'Aye, nobbut eighteen months.'

'Well, that's it. He's just too full of the joys. Plenty of good food and maybe not a lot of work to do, eh?'

'Aye, he gets good grub. Nowt but the best. And you're right – I 'aven't much work for him.'

'Well, there you are.' I held out a hand. 'Just cut down his diet and see he gets more exercise and this thing will sort itself out.'

Mr Pinkerton stared at me. 'But aren't you goin' to do anything to 'is . . . 'is . . .' Again he cast an anguished glance at our secretary.

'No, no,' I said. 'I assure you there's nothing wrong with his . . . er . . . pencil. No local trouble at all.'

I could see he was still totally unconvinced so I threw in another ploy. 'I tell you what. I'll give you some mild sedative tablets for him. They'll help a bit.'

I went through to the dispensary and counted the tablets into a box. Back in the office I handed them to the farmer with a confident smile, but his face registered only a deepening misery. Obviously I hadn't explained the thing clearly enough and as I led him along the passage to the front door I talked incessantly, putting the whole business into simple words which I was sure he would understand.

As he stood on the doorstep I gave him a final comforting pat on the shoulder and though I was almost breathless with my own babbling I thought it best to sum up the entire oration before he left.

'So there you are,' I said with a light laugh. 'Reduce his food, see that he gets plenty of work and exercise and give him one of the tablets night and morning.'

The farmer's mouth drooped until I thought he would burst into tears then he turned and trailed down the steps into the street. He took a couple of indeterminate strides then swung round and his voice rose in a plaintive wail.

'But Mr Herriot . . . 'ow about 'is pencil?'

And when little Mr Gilby crashed moaning on the cobbles of his byre floor, my first thought was that it was unfair that it should happen to him of all people.

Because the natural delicacy and reticence of the times were embodied in him to an extreme degree. Even his physical make-up had something ethereal about it; nine stones of tiny bones, taut skin with no fat and a gentle, innocent face, almost child-like despite his fifty years. Nobody had ever heard Mr Gilby swear or use a vulgar expression; in fact he was the only farmer I have ever known who talked about cow's 'manure'.

Besides, as a strict methodist he didn't drink or indulge in worldly pleasures and had never been known to tell a lie. Altogether he was so good that I would have regarded him with deep suspicion if he had been anybody else. But I had come to know Mr Gilby. He was a nice little man, he was as honest as the day. I would have trusted him with my life.

That was why I was so sad to see him lying there. It had happened so quickly. We had just come into the byre and he pointed to a black Angus Cross cow almost opposite the door.

'That's 'er. Got a touch o'cold, I think.' He knew I would want to take the temperature and grasped the tail before putting one foot across the channel so that he could slide between the cow and her neighbour. That was when it happened; when his legs were wide apart in the worst possible position.

In a way I wasn't surprised because that tail had been swishing bad-temperedly as we came in, and I am always a bit wary of black cows anyway. She didn't seem to like our sudden entry and lashed out with her right hind foot with the speed of light, catching him with her flinty hoof full in the crutch as his legs were splayed. He was wearing only frayed, much-washed overall trousers and the protection was nil.

I winced as the foot went home with an appalling thud, but Mr Gilby showed no emotion at all. He dropped as though on the receiving end of a firing squad and lay motionless on the hard stones, his hands clutched between his legs. It was only after several seconds that he began to moan softly.

As I hurried to his aid I felt it was wrong that I should be witnessing this disintegration of his modest façade. The little farmer, I was sure, would rather have died than be caught in this inelegant position, grovelling on the floor gripping frantically at an unmentionable area. I kneeled on the cobbles and patted his shoulder while he fought his inner battle with his agony.

After a while he felt well enough to sit up and I put my arm around him and supported him while perspiration bedewed the greenish pallor of his face. That was when the embarrassment began to creep in, because though he had removed his hands from their compromising position he was clearly deeply ashamed at being caught in a coarse attitude.

I felt strangely helpless. The little man couldn't relieve his feelings in the usual way by cursing the animal and fate in general, nor could I help him to laugh the thing off with a few earthy remarks. This sort of thing happens now and then in the present day and usually gives rise to a certain amount of ripe comment, often embracing the possible effect on the victim's future sex life. It all helps.

But here in Mr Gilby's byre there was only an uncomfortable silence. After a time the colour began to return to his cheeks and the little man struggled slowly to his feet. He took a couple of deep breaths then looked at me unhappily. Obviously he thought he owed me some explanation, even apology, for his tasteless behaviour.

As the minutes passed the tension rose. Mr Gilby's mouth twitched once or twice as though he were about to speak but he seemed unable to find the words. At length he appeared to come to a decision. He cleared his throat, looked around him carefully then put his lips close to my ear. He clarified the whole situation by one hoarsely whispered, deeply confidential sentence.

'Right in the privates, Mr Herriot.'

I referred earlier to the prevailing shyness about the natural functions and this did indeed give rise to problems.

One slight difficulty which all country vets encounter is that there comes a time on a long round when they have to urinate. When I first came to Yorkshire it seemed the most natural thing in the world for me to retire to a corner of a cow byre to relieve myself and it was utterly incomprehensible that anybody of my own sex should find this embarrassing. But it soon became obvious that the farmers were shuffling their feet, looking pointedly in the opposite direction or showing other signs of unease.

My attempts to laugh the incident off met with no success. Jocular remarks thrown over my shoulder like 'Just wringing out a kidney' or 'This method gives instant relief', were greeted with serious nods and mutterings of 'Aye . . . aye . . . aye . . . that's right.' I often had to resort to sneaking into some deserted outhouse as soon as I arrived, but very often the farmer would burst in and catch me in the act and retreat bashfully.

The farmers themselves added to my difficulties by their hospitable custom of pushing large mugs of tea into my hand at every opportunity. At times I shrank from causing offence in the buildings and when under stress took refuge in the open countryside. But even this was fraught with peril, because though I always selected a deserted road with the moors stretching empty to the far horizon the landscape within seconds invariably became black with cars, all driven by women and all bearing down on me at high speed.

I recall with quaking shame one occasion when a carload of middle-aged spinsters stopped and questioned me at length about the quickest way to Darrowby while a dark pool spread accusingly around my feet.

But I suppose there are exceptions to every rule, and there was one time when the reaction to my predicament was different. I had consumed my usual quota of tea and on top of this one kind chap had opened a couple of pint bottles of brown ale after a sweating session castrating calves in a tin-roofed shed. By the time I arrived at old Mr Ainsley's I was in dire straits.

But there was nobody around. I tiptoed into the byre, slunk into a corner and blessedly opened the flood gates. I was in mid flow when I heard the clatter of heavy boots on the cobbles behind me. The old man, shoulders hunched, hands in pockets, was standing there watching me.

Oh dear, it had happened again, but I wasn't going to stop now. With a sickly smile I looked over my shoulder at him.

'Sorry to make free with your cow house like this, Mr Ainsley,' I said in what I hoped was a light, bantering tone. 'But I had no option. When I have to go I just have to go. Maybe I have a weak bladder or something.'

The old man regarded me impassively for a few moments then he nodded his head several times.

'Aye, ah knaw, ah knaw,' he said gloomily. 'You're like me, Mr Herriot. Ah's allus pissin'.'

twenty-one

Little pictures kept floating up into my mind. Memories from the very early days at Skeldale House. Before the RAF, before Helen . . .

Siegfried and I were at breakfast in the big dining-room. My colleague looked up from a letter he was reading.

'James, do you remember Stewie Brannan?'

I smiled. 'I could hardly forget. That was quite a day at Brawton races.' I would always carry a vivid recollection of Siegfried's amiable college chum with me.

'Yes . . . yes, it was.' Siegfried nodded briefly. 'Well I've got a letter from him here. He's got six kids now, and though he doesn't complain, I don't think life is exactly a picnic working in a dump like Hensfield. Especially when he knocks a bare living out of it.' He pulled thoughtfully at the lobe of his ear. 'You know, James, it would be rather nice if he could have a break. Would you be willing to go through there and run his practice for a couple of weeks so that he could take his family on holiday?'

'Certainly. Glad to. But you'll be a bit pushed here on your own, won't you?'

Siegfried waved a hand. 'It'll do me good. Anyway it's the quiet time for us. I'll write back today.'

Stewie grasped the opportunity eagerly and within a few days I was on the road to Hensfield. Yorkshire is the biggest county in England and it must be the most varied. I could hardly believe it when, less than two hours after leaving the clean grassy fells and crystal air of Darrowby, I saw the forest of factory chimneys spouting from the brown pall of grime.

This was the industrial West Riding and I drove past mills as dark and satanic as any I had dreamed of, past long rows of dreary featureless houses where the workers lived. Everything was black; houses, mills, walls, trees, even the surrounding hillsides, smeared and soiled from the smoke which drifted across the town from a hundred belching stacks.

Stewie's surgery was right in the heart of it, a gloomy edifice in a terrace of sooty stone. As I rang the bell I read the painted board: 'Stewart Brannan MRCVS, Veterinary Surgeon and Canine Specialist.' I was wondering what the Royal College would think about the last part when the door opened and my colleague stood before me.

He seemed to fill the entrance. If anything he was fatter than before, but that was the only difference. Since it was August I couldn't expect him to be wearing his navy nap overcoat, but otherwise he was as I remembered him in Darrowby; the big, meaty, good-natured face, the greasy black hair slicked across the brow which always seemed to carry a gentle dew of perspiration.

He reached out, grabbed my hand and pulled me delightedly through the doorway.

'Jim! Great to see you!' He put an arm round my shoulders as we crossed a dark hallway. 'It's so good of you to help me out like this. The family are thrilled – they're all in the town shopping for the holiday. We've got fixed up in a flat at Blackpool.' His permanent smile widened.

We went into a room at the back where a rickety kitchen-type table stood on brown linoleum. I saw a sink in one corner, a few shelves with bottles and a white-painted cupboard. The atmosphere held a faint redolence of carbolic and cat's urine.

'This is where I see the animals,' Stewie said contentedly. He looked at his watch. 'Twenty past five – I have a surgery at five thirty. I'll show you round till then.'

It didn't take long because there wasn't much to see. I knew there was a more fashionable veterinary firm in Hensfield and that Stewie made his living from the poor people of the town; the whole set-up was an illustration of practice on a shoestring. There didn't seem to be more than one of anything – one straight suture needle, one curved needle, one pair of scissors, one syringe. There was a sparse selection of drugs and an extraordinary array of dispensing bottles and jars. These bottles were of many strange shapes – weird things which I had never seen in a dispensary before.

Stewie seemed to read my thoughts. 'It's nothing great, Jim. I haven't a smart practice and I don't make a lot, but we manage to clear the housekeeping and that's the main thing.'

The phrase was familiar. 'Clear the housekeeping' – that was how he had put it when I first met him at Brawton races. It seemed to be the lodestar of his life.

The end of the room was cut off by a curtain which my colleague drew to one side.

'This is what you might call the waiting room.' He smiled as I looked in some surprise at half a dozen wooden chairs arranged round the three walls. 'No high-powered stuff, Jim, no queues into the streets, but we get by.'

Some of Stewie's clients were already filing in; two little girls with a black dog, a cloth-capped old man with a terrier on a string, a teenage boy carrying a rabbit in a basket.

'Right,' the big man said. 'We'll get started,' He pulled on a white coat, opened the curtain and said, 'First, please.'

The little girls put their dog on the table. He was a long-tailed mixture of breeds and he stood trembling with fear, rolling his eyes apprehensively at the white coat.

'All right, lad,' Stewie murmured. 'I'm not going to hurt you.' He stroked and patted the quivering head before turning to the girls. 'What's the trouble, then?'

'It's 'is leg, 'e's lame,' one of them replied.

As if in confirmation the little dog raised a fore leg and held it up with a pitiful expression. Stewie engulfed the limb with his great hand and palpated it with the utmost care. And it struck me immediately – the gentleness of this shambling bear of a man.

'There's nothing broken,' he said. 'He's just sprained his shoulder. Try to rest it for a few days and rub this in night and morning.'

He poured some whitish liniment from a Winchester bottle into one of the odd-shaped bottles and handed it over.

One of the little girls held out her hand and unclasped her fingers to reveal a shilling in her palm.

'Thanks,' said Stewie without surprise. 'Goodbye.'

He saw several other cases, then as he was on his way to the curtain two grubby urchins appeared through the door at the other end of the room. They carried a clothes basket containing a widely varied assortment of glassware.

Stewie bent over the basket, lifting out HP sauce bottles, pickle jars, ketchup containers and examining them with the air of a connoisseur. At length he appeared to come to a decision.

'Threepence,' he said.

'Sixpence,' said the urchins in unison.

'Fourpence,' grunted Stewie.

'Sixpence,' chorused the urchins.

'Fivepence,' my colleague muttered doggedly.

'Sixpence!' There was a hint of triumph in the cry.

Stewie sighed. 'Go on then.' He passed over the coin and began to stack the bottles under the sink.

'I just scrape off the labels and give them a good boil up, Jim.'

'I see.'

'It's a big saving.'

'Yes, of course.' The mystery of the strangely shaped dispensing bottles was suddenly resolved.

It was six thirty when the last client came through the curtain. I had watched Stewie examining each animal carefully, taking his time and treating their conditions ably within the confines of his limited resources. His charges were all around a shilling to two shillings and it was easy to see why he only just cleared the housekeeping.

One other thing I noticed; the people all seemed to like him. He had no 'front' but he was kind and concerned. I felt there was a lesson there.

The last arrival was a stout lady with a prim manner and a very correct manner of speech.

'My dog was bit last week,' she announced, 'and I'm afraid the wound is goin' antiseptic.'

'Ah yes.' Stewie nodded gravely. The banana fingers explored the tumefied area on the animal's neck with a gossamer touch. 'It's quite nasty, really. He could have an abscess there if we're not careful.'

He took a long time over clipping the hair away, swabbing out the deep puncture with peroxide of hydrogen. Then he puffed in some dusting powder, applied a pad of cotton wool and secured it with a bandage. He followed with an anti-staphylococcal injection and finally handed over a sauce bottle filled to the rim with acriflavine solution.

'Use as directed on the label,' he said, then stood back as the lady opened her purse expectantly.

A long inward struggle showed in the occasional twitches of his cheeks and flickerings of his eyelids but finally he squared his shoulders.

'That,' he said resolutely, 'will be three and sixpence.'

It was a vast fee by Stewie's standards, but probably the minimum in other veterinary establishments, and I couldn't see how he could make any profit from the transaction.

As the lady left, a sudden uproar broke out within the house. Stewie gave me a seraphic smile.

'That'll be Meg and the kids. Come and meet them.'

We went out to the hall and into an incredible hubbub. Children shouted, screamed and laughed, spades and pails clattered, a large ball thumped from wall to wall and above it all a baby bawled relentlessly.

Stewie moved into the mob and extracted a small woman.

'This,' he murmured with quiet pride, 'is my wife.' He gazed at her like a small boy admiring a film star.

'How do you do,' I said.

Meg Brannan took my hand and smiled. Any glamour about her existed only in her husband's eye. A ravaged prettiness still remained but her face bore the traces of some tough years. I could imagine her life of mother, housewife, cook, secretary, receptionist and animal nurse.

'Oh, Mr Herriot, it is good of you and Mr Farnon to help us out like this. We're so looking forward to going away.' Her eyes held a faintly desperate gleam but they were kind.

I shrugged. 'Oh it's a pleasure, Mrs Brannan. I'm sure I'll enjoy it and I hope you all have a marvellous holiday.' I really meant it – she looked as though she needed one.

I was introduced to the children but I never really got them sorted out. Apart from the baby, who yelled indefatigably from leather lungs, I think there were three little boys and two little girls, but I couldn't be sure – they moved around too quickly.

The only time they were silent was for a brief period at supper when Meg fed them and us from a kind of cauldron in which floated chunks of mutton, potatoes and carrots. It was very good, too, and was followed by a vast blancmange with jam on top.

The tumult broke out again very soon as the youngsters raced through their meal and began to play in the room. One thing I found disconcerting was that two biggest boys kept throwing a large, new, painted ball from one to the other across the table as we ate. The parents said nothing about it – Meg, I felt, because she had stopped caring, and Stewie because he never had cared.

Only once when the ball whizzed past my nose and almost carried away a poised spoonful of blancmange did their father remonstrate.

'Now then, now then,' he murmured absently, and the throwing was re-sited more towards the middle of the table.

Next morning I saw the family off. Stewie had changed his dilapidated Austin Seven for a large rust-encrusted Ford V Eight. Seated at the wheel he waved and beamed through the cracked side windows with serene contentment. Meg, by his side, managed a harassed smile and at the other windows an assortment of dogs and children fought for a vantage point. As the car moved away a pram, several suitcases and a cot swayed perilously on the roof, the children yelled, the dogs barked, the baby bawled, then they were gone.

As I re-entered the house the unaccustomed silence settled around me, and with the silence came a faint unease. I had to look after this practice for two weeks and the memory of the thinly furnished surgery was not reassuring. I just didn't have the tools to tackle any major problem.

But it was easy to comfort myself. From what I had seen this wasn't the sort of place where dramatic things happened. Stewie had once said he made most of his living by castrating tom cats and I supposed if you threw in a few ear cankers and minor ailments that would be about it.

The morning surgery seemed to confirm this impression; a few humble folk led in nondescript pets with mild conditions and I happily dispensed a series of Bovril bottles and meat paste jars containing Stewie's limited drug store.

I had only one difficulty and that was with the table, which kept collapsing when I lifted the animals on to it. For some obscure reason it had folding legs held by metal struts underneath and these were apt to disengage at crucial moments, causing the patient to slide abruptly to the floor. After a while I got the hang of the thing and kept one leg jammed against the struts throughout the examination.

It was about 10.30 a.m. when I finally parted the curtains and found the waiting room empty and only the distinctive cat–dog smell lingering on the air. As I locked the door it struck me that I had very little to do till the afternoon surgery. At Darrowby I would have been dashing out to start the long day's driving round the countryside, but here almost all the work was done at the practice house.

I was wondering how I would put the time in after the single outside visit on the book when the door bell rang. Then it rang again followed by a frantic pounding on the wood. I hurried through the curtain and turned the handle. A well dressed young couple stood on the step. The man held a Golden Labrador in his arms and behind them a caravan drawn by a large gleaming car stood by the kerb.

'Are you the vet?' the girl gasped. She was in her twenties, auburn haired, extremely attractive, but her eyes were terrified.

I nodded. 'Yes – yes, I am. What's the trouble?'

'It's our dog.' The young man's voice was hoarse, his face deathly pale. 'A car hit him.'

I glanced over the motionless yellow form. 'Is he badly hurt?'

There were a few moments of silence then the girl spoke almost in a whisper. 'Look at his hind leg.'

I stepped forward and as I peered into the crook of the

man's arm a freezing wave drove through me. The limb was hanging off at the hock. Not fractured but snapped through the joint and dangling from what looked like a mere shred of skin. In the bright morning sunshine the white ends of naked bones glittered with a sickening lustre.

It seemed a long time before I came out of my first shock and found myself staring stupidly at the animal. And when I spoke the voice didn't sound like my own.

'Bring him in,' I muttered, and as I led the way back through the odorous waiting room the realization burst on me that I had been wrong when I thought that nothing ever happened here.

twenty-two

I held the curtains apart as the young man staggered in and placed his burden on the table.

Now I could see the whole thing; the typical signs of a road accident; the dirt driven savagely into the glossy gold of the coat, the multiple abrasions. But that mangled leg wasn't typical. I had never seen anything like it before.

I dragged my eyes round to the girl. 'How did it happen?'

'Oh, just in a flash.' The tears welled in her eyes. 'We are on a caravanning holiday. We had no intention of staying in Hensfield' – (I could understand that) – 'but we stopped for a newspaper, Kim jumped out of the car and that was it.'

I looked at the big dog stretched motionless on the table. I reached out a hand and gently ran my fingers over the noble outlines of the head.

'Poor old lad,' I murmured and for an instant the beautiful hazel eyes turned to me and the tail thumped briefly against the wood.

'Where have you come from?' I asked.

'Surrey,' the young man replied. He looked rather like the

prosperous young stockbroker that the name conjured up.

I rubbed my chin. 'I see . . .' A way of escape shone for a moment in the tunnel. 'Perhaps if I patch him up you could get him back to your own vet there.'

He looked at his wife for a moment then back at me. 'And what would they do there? Amputate his leg?'

I was silent. If an animal in this condition arrived in one of those high-powered southern practices with plenty of skilled assistance and full surgical equipment that's what they probably would do. It would be the only sensible thing.

The girl broke in on my thoughts. 'Anyway, if it's at all possible to save his leg something has to be done right now. Isn't that so?' She gazed at me appealingly.

'Yes,' I said huskily. 'That's right.' I began to examine the dog. The abrasions on the skin were trivial. He was shocked but his mucous membranes were pink enough to suggest that there was no internal haemorrhage. He had escaped serious injury except for that terrible leg.

I stared at it intently, appalled by the smooth glistening articular surfaces of the tibio-tarsal joint. There was something obscene in its exposure in a living animal. It was as though the hock had been broken open by brutal inquisitive hands.

I began a feverish search of the premises, pulling open drawers, cupboards, opening tins and boxes. My heart leaped at each little find; a jar of catgut in spirit, a packet of lint, a sprinkler tin of iodoform, and – treasure trove indeed – a bottle of barbiturate anaesthetic.

Most of all I needed antibiotics, but it was pointless looking for those because they hadn't been discovered yet. But I did hope fervently for just an ounce or two of sulphanilamide. and there I was disappointed, because Stewie's menage didn't stretch to that. It was when I came upon the box of plaster of paris bandages that something seemed to click.

At that time in the late thirties the Spanish civil war was vivid in people's minds. In the chaos of the later stages there had been no proper medicaments to treat the terrible wounds. They had often been encased in plaster and left, in the grim phrase, to 'stew in their own juice'. Sometimes the results were surprisingly good.

I grabbed the bandages. I knew what I was going to do. Gripped by a fierce determination I inserted the needle into the radial vein and slowly injected the anaesthetic. Kim blinked, yawned lazily and went to sleep. I quickly laid out my meagre armoury then began to shift the dog into a better position. But I had forgotten about the table and as I lifted the hind quarters the whole thing gave way and the dog slithered helplessly towards the floor.

'Catch him!' At my frantic shout the man grabbed the inert form, then I reinserted the slots in their holes and got the wooden surface back on the level.

'Put your leg under there,' I gasped, then turned to the girl. 'And would you please do the same at the other end. This table mustn't fall over once I get started.'

Silently they complied and as I looked at them, each with a leg jammed against the underside, I felt a deep sense of shame. What sort of place did they think this was?

But for a long time after I forgot everything. First I put the joint back in place, slipping the ridges of the tibial-tarsal trochlea into the grooves at the distal end of the tibia as I had done so often in the anatomy lab at college. And I noticed with a flicker of hope that some of the ligaments were still intact and, most important, that a few good blood vessels still ran down to the lower part of the limb.

I never said a word as I cleaned and disinfected the area, puffed iodoform into every crevice and began to stitch. I stitched interminably, pulling together shattered tendons, torn joint capsule and fascia. It was a warm morning and as the sun beat on the surgery window the sweat broke out on my forehead. By the time I had sutured the skin a little river was flowing down my nose and dripping from the tip. Next, more iodoform, then the lint and finally two of the plaster bandages, making a firm cast above the hock down over the foot.

I straightened up and faced the young couple. They had never moved from their uncomfortable postures as they held the table upright but I gazed at them as though seeing them for the first time.

I mopped my brow and drew a long breath. 'Well, that's it. I'd be inclined to leave it as it is for a week, then wherever you are let a vet have a look at it.'

They were silent for a moment then the girl spoke. 'I would rather you saw it yourself.' Her husband nodded agreement.

'Really?' I was amazed. I had thought they would never want to see me, my smelly waiting room or my collapsible table again.

'Yes, of course we would,' the man said. 'You have taken such pains over him. Whatever happens we are deeply grateful to you, Mr Brannan.'

'Oh, I'm not Mr Brannan, he's on holiday. I'm his locum, my name is Herriot.'

He held out his hand. 'Well thank you again, Mr Herriot. I am Peter Gillard and this is my wife. Marjorie.'

We shook hands and he took the dog in his arms and went out to the car.

For the next few days I couldn't keep Kim's leg out of my mind. At times I felt I was crazy trying to salvage a limb that was joined to the dog only by a strip of skin. I had never met anything remotely like it before and in unoccupied moments that hock joint with all its imponderables would float across my vision.

There were plenty of these moments because Stewie's was a restful practice. Apart from the three daily surgeries there was little activity, and in particular the uncomfortable pre-breakfast call so common in Darrowby was unknown here.

The Brannans had left the house and me in the care of Mrs Holroyd, an elderly widow of raddled appearance who slouched around in a flowered overall down which ash cascaded from a permanently dangling cigarette. She wasn't a good riser but she soon had me trained, because after a few mornings when I couldn't find her I began to prepare my own breakfast and that was how it stayed.

However, at other times she looked after me very well. She was what you might call a good rough cook and pushed large tasty meals at me regularly with a 'There y'are, luv,' watching me impassively till I started to eat. The only thing that disturbed me was the long trembling finger of ash which always hung over my food from the cigarette that was part of her.

Mrs Holroyd also took telephone messages when I wasn't around. There weren't many outside visits but two have stuck in my memory.

The first was when I looked on the pad and read, 'Go to Mr Pimmarov to see bulldog,' in Mrs Holroyd's careful back-sloped script.

'Pimmarov?' I asked her. 'Was he a Russian gentleman?'

'Dunno, luv, never asked 'im.'

'Well – did he sound foreign? I mean did he speak broken English?'

'Nay, luv, Yorkshire as me, 'e were.'

'Ah well, never mind, Mrs Holroyd. What's his address?'

She gave me a surprised look. 'How should ah know? He never said.'

'But . . . but Mrs Holroyd. How can I visit him when I don't know where he lives?'

'Well you'll know best about that, luv.'

I was baffled. 'But he must have told you.'

'Now then, young man, Pimmarov was all 'e told me. Said you would know.' She stuck out her chin, her cigarette quivered and she regarded me stonily. Maybe she had had similar sessions with Stewie, but she left me in no doubt that the interview was over.

During the day I tried not to think about it but the knowledge that somewhere in the neighbourhood there was an ailing bulldog that I could not succour was worrying. I just hoped it was nothing fatal.

A phone call at 7 p.m. resolved my fears.

'Is that t'vet?' The voice was gruff and grumpy.

'Yes . . . speaking.'

'Well, ah've been waitin' all day for tha. When are you comin' to see ma flippin' bulldog?'

A light glimmered. But still . . . that accent . . . no suggestion of the Kremlin . . . not a hint of the Steppes.

'Oh, I'm terribly sorry,' I gabbled. 'I'm afraid there's been a little misunderstanding. I'm doing Mr Brannan's work and I don't know the district. I do hope your dog isn't seriously ill.'

'Nay, nay, nobbut a bit o' cough, but ah want 'im seein' to.'

'Certainly, certainly, I'll be right out, Mr . . . er . . .'

'Pym's ma name and ah live next to t'post office in Roff village.'

'Roff?'

'Aye, two miles outside Hensfield.'

I sighed with relief. 'Very good, Mr Pym, I'm on my way.'

'Thank ye.' The voice sounded mollified. 'Well, tha knows me now, don't tha – Pym o' Roff.'

The light was blinding. 'Pym o' Roff!' Such a simple explanation.

A lot of Mrs Holroyd's messages were eccentric but I could usually interpret them after some thought. However one bizarre entry jolted me later in the week. It read simply: 'Johnson, 12, Back Lane, Smiling Harry Syphilis.'

I wrestled with this for a long time before making a diffident approach to Mrs Holroyd.

She was kneading dough for scones and didn't look up as I entered the kitchen.

'Ah, Mrs Holroyd.' I rubbed my hands nervously. 'I see you have written down that I have to go to Mr Johnson's.'

'That's right, luv.'

'Well, er . . . fine, but I don't quite understand the other part – the Smiling Harry Syphilis.'

She shot a sidelong glance at me. 'Well that's 'ow you spell that word, isn't it? Ah looked it up once in a doctor's book in our 'ouse,' she said defensively.

'Oh yes, of course, yes, you've spelled it correctly. It's just the Smiling . . . and the Harry.'

Her eyes glinted dangerously and she blew a puff of smoke at me. 'Well, that's what t'feller said. Repeated it three times. Couldn't make no mistake.'

'I see. But did he mention any particular animal?'

'Naw, 'e didn't. That was what 'e said. That and no more.'
A grey spicule of ash toppled into the basin and was immediately incorporated in the scones. 'Ah do ma best, tha knows!'

'Of course you do, Mrs Holroyd,' I said hastily. 'I'll just pop round to Back Lane now.'

And Mr Johnson put everything right within seconds as he led me to a shed on his allotment.

'It's me pig, guvnor. Covered wi' big red spots. Reckon it's swine erysipelas.'

Only he pronounced it arrysipelas and he did have a slurring mode of speech. I really couldn't blame Mrs Holroyd.

Little things like that enlivened the week but the tension still mounted as I awaited the return of Kim. And even when the seventh day came round I was still in suspense because the Gillards did not appear at the morning surgery. When they failed to show up at the afternoon session I began to conclude that they had had the good sense to return south to a more sophisticated establishment. But at five thirty they were there.

I knew it even before I pulled the curtains apart. The smell of doom was everywhere, filling the premises, and when I went through the curtains it hit me; the sickening stink of putrefaction.

Gangrene. It was the fear which had haunted me all week and now it was realized.

There were about half a dozen other people in the waiting room, all keeping as far away as possible from the young couple who looked up at me with strained smiles. Kim tried to rise when he saw me but I had eyes only for the dangling useless hind limb where my once stone-hard plaster hung in sodden folds.

Of course it had to happen that the Gillards were last in and I was forced to see all the other animals first. I examined them and prescribed treatment in a stupor of misery and shame. What had I done to that beautiful dog out there? I had been crazy to try that experiment. A gangrenous leg

187

meant that even amputation might be too late to save his life. Death from septicaemia was likely now and what the hell could I do for him in this ramshackle surgery?

When at last it was their turn the Gillards came in with Kim limping between them, and it was an extra stab to realize afresh what a handsome animal he was. I bent over the great golden head and for a moment the friendly eyes looked into mine and the tail waved.

'Right,' I said to Peter Gillard, putting my arms under the chest. 'You take the back end and we'll lift him up.'

As we hoisted the heavy dog on to the table the flimsy structure disintegrated immediately, but this time the young people were ready for it and thrust their legs under the struts like a well-trained team till the surface was level again.

With Kim stretched on his side I fingered the bandage. It usually took time and patience with a special saw to remove a plaster but this was just a stinking pulp. My hand shook as I cut the bandage lengthways with scissors and removed it.

I had steeled myself against the sight of the cold dead limb with its green flesh but though there was pus and serous fluid everywhere the exposed flesh was a surprising, healthy pink. I took the foot in my hand and my heart gave a great bound. It was warm and so was the leg, right up to the hock. There was no gangrene.

Feeling suddenly weak I leaned against the table. 'I'm sorry about the terrible smell. All the pus and discharge have been decomposing under the bandage for a week but despite the mess it's not as bad as I feared.'

'Do you . . . do you think you can save his leg?' Marjorie Gillard's voice trembled.

'I don't know. I honestly don't know. So much has to happen. But I'd say it was a case of so far so good.'

I cleaned the area thoroughly with spirit, gave a dusting of iodoform and applied fresh lint and two more plaster bandages.

'You'll feel a lot more comfortable now, Kim,' I said, and the big dog flapped his tail against the wood at the sound of his name.

I turned to his owners. 'I want him to have another week in plaster, so what would you like to do?'

'Oh, we'll stay around Hensfield,' Peter Gillard replied. 'We've found a place for our caravan by the river – it's not too bad.'

'Very well, till next Saturday, then.' I watched Kim hobble out, holding his new white cast high, and as I went back into the house relief flowed over me in a warm wave.

But at the back of my mind the voice of caution sounded. There was still a long way to go . . .

twenty-three

The second week went by without incident. I had a mildly indecent postcard from Stewie and a view of Blackpool Tower from his wife. The weather was scorching and they were having the best holiday of their lives. I tried to picture them enjoying themselves but I had to wait a few weeks for the evidence – a snap taken by a beach photographer. The whole family were standing in the sea, grinning delightedly into the camera as the wavelets lapped round their ankles. The children brandished buckets and spades, the baby dangled bandy legs towards the water, but it was Stewie who fascinated me. A smile of blissful contentment beamed from beneath a knotted handkerchief, sturdy braces supported baggy flannel trousers rolled decorously calf high. He was the archetype of the British father on holiday.

The last event of my stay in Hensfield was a visit to the local greyhound track. Stewie had an appointment there every other Friday to inspect the dogs.

The Hensfield stadium was not prepossessing from the outside. It had been built in a natural hollow in the sooty hills and was surrounded by ramshackle hoardings.

It was a cool night and as I drove down to the entrance I could hear the tinny blaring from the loudspeakers. It was George Formby singing 'When I'm Cleaning Windows' and strumming on his famous ukelele.

There are all kinds of greyhound tracks. My own experience had been as a student, accompanying vets who officiated under the auspices of the National Greyhound Racing Club, but this was an unlicensed or 'flapping' track, and vastly different. I know there are many highly reputable flapping tracks but this one had a seedy air. It was, I thought wryly, just the sort of place that would be under the care of Stewie.

First I had to go to the manager's office. Mr Coker was a hard-eyed man in a shiny pin-striped suit and he nodded briefly before giving me a calculating stare.

'Your duties here are just a formality,' he said, twisting his features into a smile. 'There'll be nothing to trouble you.'

I had the impression that he was assessing me with quiet satisfaction, looking me up and down, taking in my rumpled jacket and slacks, savouring my obvious youth and inexperience. He kept the smile going as he stubbed out his cigar. 'Well, I hope you'll have a pleasant evening.'

'Thank you,' I replied, and left.

I met the judge, timekeeper and other officials then went down to a long glass-fronted bar overlooking the track. Quite suddenly I felt I was in an alien environment. The place was rapidly filling up and the faces around me were out of a different mould from the wholesome rural countenances of Darrowby. There seemed to be a large proportion of fat men in camel coats with brassy blondes in tow. Shifty-looking characters studied race cards and glared intently at the flickering numbers on the tote board.

I looked at my watch. It was time to inspect the dogs for the first race. 'When I'm cleanin' winders!' bawled George Formby as I made my way round the edge of the track to the paddock, a paved enclosure with a wire-netting surround. Five dogs were being led round the perimeter and I stood in the centre and watched them for a minute or two. Then I halted them and went from one to the other, looking at their eyes, examining their mouths for salivation and finally palpating their abdomens.

They all appeared bright and normal except number four which seemed rather full in the stomach region. A greyhound should only have a light meal on the morning of a race and nothing thereafter and I turned to the man who was holding the animal.

'Has this dog been fed within the last hour or two?' I asked.

'No,' he replied. 'He's had nothing since breakfast.'

As I passed my fingers over the abdomen again I had the feeling that several of the onlookers were watching me with unusual intentness. But I dismissed it as imagination and passed on to the next animal.

Number four was second favourite but from the moment it left its trap it was flagging. It finished last and from the darkness on the far side of the track a storm of booing broke out. I was able to make out some of the remarks which came across on the night air. 'Open your bloody eyes, vet!' was one of them. And here, in the long, brightly lit bar I could see people nudging each other and looking at me.

I felt a thrill of anger. Maybe some of those gentlemen down there thought they could cash in on Stewie's absence. I probably looked a soft touch to them.

My next visit to the paddock was greeted with friendly nods and grins from all sides. In fact there was a strong atmosphere of joviality. When I went round the dogs all was well until I came to number five and this time I couldn't be mistaken. Under my probing fingers the stomach bulged tensely and the animal gave a soft grunt as I squeezed.

'You'll have to take this dog out of the race,' I said. 'He's got a full stomach.'

The owner was standing by the kennel lad.

'Can't 'ave!' he burst out. 'He's had nowt!'

I straightened up and looked him full in the face but his eyes were reluctant to meet mine. I knew some of the tricks; a couple of pounds of steak before the race; a bowlful of bread crumbs and two pints of milk – the crumbs swelled beautifully within a short time.

'Would you like me to vomit him?' I began to move away. 'I've got some washing soda in my car – we'll soon find out.'

The man held up a hand. 'Naw, naw, I don't want you messin' about with me dog.' He gave me a malevolent glare and trailed sulkily away.

I had only just got back to the bar when I heard the announcement over the loudspeakers. 'Will the vet please report to the manager's office.'

Mr Coker looked up from his desk and glared at me through a haze of cigar smoke. 'You've taken a dog out of the race!'

'That's right, I'm sorry, but his stomach was full.'

'But damn it . . . !' He stabbed a finger at me then subsided and forced a tortured smile across his face. 'Now, Mr Herriot, we have to be reasonable in these matters. I've no doubt you know your job, but don't you think there's just a chance you could be wrong?' He waved his cigar expansively. 'After all, anybody can make a mistake, so perhaps you would be kind enough to reconsider.' He stretched his smile wider.

'No, I'm sorry, Mr Coker, but that would be impossible.'

There was a long pause. 'That's your last word, then?'

'It is.'

The smile vanished and he gave me a threatening stare.

'Now look,' he said. 'You've mucked up that race and it's a serious matter. I don't want any repetition, do you understand?' He ground his cigar out savagely and his jaw jutted. 'So I hope we won't have any more trouble like this.'

'I hope so, too, Mr Coker,' I said as I went out.

It seemed a long way down to the paddock on my next visit. It was very dark now and I was conscious of the hum of the crowd, the shouts of the bookies and George and his ukelele still going full blast. 'Oh, don't the wind blow cold!' he roared.

This time it was dog number two. I could feel the tension as I examined him and found the same turgid belly.

'This one's out,' I said, and apart from a few black looks there was no argument.

They say bad news travels fast and I had hardly started my

return journey when George was switched off and the loud-speaker asked me to report to the manager's office.

Mr Coker was no longer at his desk. He was pacing up and down agitatedly and when he saw me he did another length of the room before coming to a halt. His expression was venomous and it was clear he had decided that the tough approach was best.

'What the bloody hell do you think you're playing at?' he barked. 'Are you trying to ruin this meeting?'

'No,' I replied. 'I've just taken out another dog which was unfit to run. That's my job. That's what I'm here for.'

His face flushed deep red. 'I don't think you know what you're here for. Mr Brannan goes off on holiday and leaves us at the mercy of a young clever clogs like you, throwing your weight about and spoiling people's pleasure. Wait till I see him!'

'Mr Brannan would have done just the same as I have. Any veterinary surgeon would.'

'Rubbish! Don't tell me what it's all about – you're still wet behind the ears.' He advanced slowly towards me. 'But I'll tell you this, I've had enough! So get it straight, once and for all – no more of this nonsense. Cut it out!'

I felt my heart thudding as I went down to see the dogs for the next race. As I examined the five animals the owners and kennel lads fixed me with a hypnotic stare as though I were some strange freak. My pulse began to slow down when I found there were no full stomachs this time and I glanced back in relief along the line. I was about to walk away when I noticed that number one looked a little unusual. I went back and bent over him, trying to decide what it was about him that had caught my attention. Then I realized what it was – he looked sleepy. The head was hanging slightly and he had an air of apathy.

I lifted his chin and looked into his eyes. The pupils were dilated and every now and then there was a faint twitch of nystagmus. There was absolutely no doubt about it – he had received some kind of sedative. He had been doped.

The men in the paddock were very still as I stood upright.

For a few moments I gazed through the wire netting at the brightly lit green oval, feeling the night air cold on my cheeks. George was still at it on the loudspeakers.

'Oh Mr Wu,' he trilled. 'What can I do?'

Well I knew what I had to do, anyway. I tapped the dog on the back.

'This one's out,' I said.

I didn't wait for the announcement and was half way up the steps to the manager's office before I heard the request for my presence blared across the stadium.

When I opened the door I half expected Mr Coker to rush at me and attack me and I was surprised when I found him sitting at his desk, his head buried in his hands. I stood there on the carpet for some time before he raised a ghastly countenance to me.

'Is it true?' he whispered despairingly. 'Have you done it again?'

I nodded. 'Afraid so.'

His lips trembled but he didn't say anything, and after a brief, disbelieving scrutiny he sank his head in his hands again.

I waited for a minute or two but when he stayed like that, quite motionless, I realized that the audience was at an end and took my leave.

I found no fault with the dogs for the next race and as I left the paddock an unaccustomed peace settled around me. I couldn't understand it when I heard the loudspeaker again – 'Will the vet please report . . .' But this time it was to the paddock and I wondered if a dog had been injured. Anyway, it would be a relief to do a bit of real vetting for a change.

But when I arrived there were no animals to be seen; only two men cradling a fat companion in their arms.

'What's this?' I asked one of them.

'Ambrose 'ere fell down the steps in the stand and skinned 'is knee.'

I stared at him. 'But I'm a vet, not a doctor.'

'Ain't no doctor on the track,' the man mumbled. 'We reckoned you could patch 'im up.'

Ah well, it was a funny night. 'Put him over on that bench,' I said.

I rolled up the trouser to reveal a rather revolting fat dimpled knee. Ambrose emitted a hollow groan as I touched a very minor abrasion on the patella.

'It's nothing much,' I said. 'You've just knocked a bit of skin off.'

Ambrose looked at me tremblingly. 'Aye, but it could go t'wrong way, couldn't it? I don't want no blood poisonin'.'

'All right, I'll put something on it.' I looked inside Stewie's medical bag. The selection was limited but I found some tincture of iodine and I poured a little on a pad of cotton wool and dabbed the wound.

Ambrose gave a shrill yelp. 'Bloody 'ell, that 'urts! What are you doin' to me?' His foot jerked up and rapped me sharply on the elbow.

Even my human patients kicked me, it seemed. I smiled reassuringly. 'Don't worry, it won't sting for long. I'll put a bandage on now.'

I bound up the knee, rolled down the trouser and patted the fat man's shoulder. 'There you are – good as new.'

He got off the bench, nodded, then grimacing painfully, prepared to leave. But an afterthought appeared to strike him and he pulled a handful of change from his pocket. He rummaged among it with a forefinger before selecting a coin which he pressed into my palm.

'There y'are,' he said.

I looked at the coin. It was a sixpence, the fee for my only piece of doctoring of my own species. I stared stupidly at it for a long time and when I finally looked up with the half-formed idea of throwing Ambrose's honorarium back at his head the man was limping into the crowd and was soon lost to sight.

Back in the bar I was gazing apathetically through the glass at the dogs parading round the track when I felt a hand on my arm. I turned and recognized a man I had spotted earlier in the evening. He was one of a group of three men and three women, the men dark, tight-suited, foreign-looking, the women loud and over-dressed. There was something sinister about them and I remembered thinking they could have passed without question as members of the Mafia.

The man put his face close to mine and I had a brief impression of black, darting eyes and a predatory smile.

'Is number three fit?' he whispered.

I couldn't understand the question. He seemed to know I was the vet and surely it was obvious that if I had passed the dog I considered him fit.

'Yes,' I replied. 'Yes, he is.'

The man nodded vigorously and gave me a knowing glance from hooded eyes. He returned and held a short, intimate conversation with his friends, then they all turned and looked over at me approvingly.

I was bewildered, then it struck me that they may have thought I was giving them an inside tip. To this day I am not really sure but I think that was it because when number three finished nowhere in the race their attitude changed dramatically and they flashed me some black glares which made them look more like the Mafia than ever.

Anyway I had no more trouble down at the paddock for the rest of the evening. No more dogs to take out, which was just as well, because I had made enough enemies for one night.

After the last race I looked around the long bar. Most of the tables were occupied by people having a final drink, but I noticed an empty one and sank wearily into a chair. Stewie had asked me to stay for half an hour after the finish to make sure all the dogs got away safely and I would stick to my bargain even though what I wanted most in the world was to get away from here and never come back.

George was still in splendid voice on the loudspeakers. 'I always get to bed by half past nine,' he warbled, and I felt strongly that he had a point there.

Along the bar counter were assembled most of the people with whom I had clashed; Mr Coker and other officials and dog owners. There was a lot of nudging and whispering and I didn't have to be told the subject of their discussion. The

Mafia, too, were doing their bit with fierce side glances and I could almost feel the waves of antagonism beating against me.

My gloomy thoughts were interrupted by the arrival of a bookie and his clerk. The bookie dropped into a chair opposite me and tipped out a huge leather bag on to the table. I had never seen so much money in my life. I peered at the man over a mountain of fivers and pounds and ten-shilling notes while little streams and tributaries of coins ran down its flanks.

The two of them began a methodical stacking and counting of the loot while I watched hypnotically. They had eroded the mountain to about half its height when the bookie caught my eye. Maybe he thought I looked envious or poverty-stricken or just miserable because he put his finger behind a stray half crown and flicked it expertly across the smooth surface in my direction.

'Get yourself a drink, son,' he said.

It was the second time I had been offered money during the last hour and I was almost as much taken aback as the first time. The bookie looked at me expressionlessly for a moment then he grinned. He had an attractively ugly, good-natured face that I liked instinctively and suddenly I felt grateful to him, not for the money but for the sight of a friendly face. It was the only one I had seen all evening.

I smiled back. 'Thanks,' I said. I lifted the half crown and went over to the bar.

I awoke next morning with the knowledge that it was my last day at Hensfield. Stewie was due back at lunch time.

When I parted the now familiar curtains at the morning surgery I still felt a vague depression, a hangover from my unhappy night at the dog track.

But when I looked into the waiting room my mood lightened immediately. There was only one animal among the odd assortment of chairs but that animal was Kim, massive, golden and beautiful, sitting between his owners, and when he saw me he sprang up with swishing tail and laughing mouth.

There was none of the smell which had horrified me before but as I looked at the dog I could sniff something else – the sweet, sweet scent of success. Because he was touching the ground with that leg; not putting any weight on it but definitely dotting it down as he capered around me.

In an instant I was back in my world again and Mr Coker and the events of last night were but the dissolving mists of a bad dream.

I could hardly wait to get started.

'Get him on the table,' I cried, then began to laugh as the Gillards automatically pushed their legs against the collapsible struts. They knew the drill now.

I had to restrain myself from doing a dance of joy when I got the plaster off. There was a bit of discharge but when I cleaned it away I found healthy granulation tissue everywhere. Pink new flesh binding the shattered joint together, smoothing over and hiding the original mutilation.

'Is his leg safe now?' Marjorie Gillard asked softly.

I looked at her and smiled. 'Yes, it is. There's no doubt about it now.' I rubbed my hand under the big dog's chin and the tail beat ecstatically on the wood. 'He'll probably have a stiff joint but that won't matter, will it?'

I applied the last of Stewie's bandages then we hoisted Kim off the table.

'Well, that's it,' I said. 'Take him to your own vet in another fortnight. After that I don't think he'll need a bandage at all.'

The Gillards left on their journey back to the south and a couple of hours later Stewie and his family returned. The children were very brown; even the baby, still bawling resolutely, had a fine tan. The skin had peeled off Meg's nose but she looked wonderfully relaxed. Stewie, in open necked shirt and with a face like a boiled lobster, seemed to have put on weight.

'That holiday saved our lives, Jim,' he said. 'I can't thank you enough, and please tell Siegfried how grateful we are.' He looked fondly at his turbulent brood flooding through the house, then as an afterthought he turned to me.

'Is everything all right in the practice?'

'Yes, Stewie, it is. I had my ups and downs of course.'

He laughed. 'Don't we all.'

'We certainly do, but everything's fine now.'

And everything did seem fine as I drove away from the smoke. I watched the houses thin and fall away behind me till the whole world opened out clean and free and I saw the green line of the fells rising over Darrowby.

I suppose we all tend to remember the good things but as it turned out I had no option. The following Christmas I had a letter from the Gillards with a packet of snapshots showing a big golden dog clearing a gate, leaping high for a ball, strutting proudly with a stick in his mouth. There was hardly any stiffness in the leg, they said; he was perfectly sound.

So even now when I think of Hensfield the thing I remember best is Kim.

twenty-four

There was a lot of shouting in the RAF. The NCOs always seemed to be shouting at me or at somebody else and a lot of them had impressively powerful voices. But for sheer volume I don't think any of them could beat Len Hampson.

I was on the way to Len's farm and on an impulse I pulled up the car and leaned for a moment on the wheel. It was a hot still day in late summer and this was one of the softer corners of the Dales, sheltered by the enclosing fells from the harsh winds which shrivelled all but the heather and the tough moorland grass.

Here, great trees, oak, elm and sycamore in full rich leaf, stood in gentle majesty in the green dips and hollows, their branches quite still in the windless air.

In all the grassy miles around me I could see no movement, nor could I hear anything except the fleeting hum of a bee and the distant bleating of a sheep.

Through the open window drifted the scents of summer; warm grass, clover and the sweetness of hidden flowers. But in the car they had to compete with the all-pervading smell of cow. I had spent the last hour injecting fifty wild cattle and I sat there in soiled breeches and sweat-soaked shirt looking out sleepily at the tranquil landscape.

I opened the door and Sam jumped out and trotted into a nearby wood. I followed him into the cool shade, into the damp secret fragrance of pine needles and fallen leaves which came from the dark heart of the crowding boles. From somewhere in the branches high above I could hear that most soothing of sounds, the cooing of a woodpigeon.

Then, although the farm was two fields away, I heard Len Hampson's voice. He wasn't calling the cattle home or anything like that. He was just conversing with his family as he always did in a long tireless shout.

I drove on to the farm and he opened the gate to let me into the yard.

'Good morning, Mr Hampson,' I said.

'NOW THEN, MR HERRIOT,' he bawled. 'IT'S A GRAND MORNIN'.'

The blast of sound drove me back a step but his three sons smiled contentedly. No doubt they were used to it.

I stayed at a safe distance. 'You want me to see a pig.'

'AYE, A GOOD BACON PIG. GONE RIGHT OFF. IT HASN'T ATE NOWT FOR TWO DAYS.'

We went into the pig pen and it was easy to pick out my patient. Most of the big white occupants careered around at the sight of a stranger, but one of them stood quietly in a corner.

It isn't often a pig will stand unresisting as you take its temperature but this one never stirred as I slipped the thermometer into its rectum. There was only a slight fever but the animal had the look of doom about it; back slightly arched, unwilling to move, eyes withdrawn and anxious.

I looked up at Len Hampson's red-faced bulk leaning over the wall of the pen.

'Did this start suddenly or gradually?' I asked.

'RIGHT SUDDEN!' In the confined space the full throated yell was deafening. 'HE WERE AS RIGHT AS NINEPENCE ON MONDAY NIGHT AND LIKE THIS ON TUESDAY MORNIN'.'

I felt my way over the pig's abdomen. The musculature was tense and boardlike and the abdominal contents were difficult to palpate because of this, but the whole area was tender to the touch.

'I've seen them like this before,' I said. 'This pig has a ruptured bowel. They do it when they are fighting or jostling each other, especially when they are full after a meal.'

'WHAT'S GOIN' TO 'APPEN THEN?'

'Well, the food material has leaked into the abdomen, causing peritonitis. I've opened up pigs like this and they are a mass of adhesions – the abdominal organs all growing together. I'm afraid the chances of recovery are very small.'

He took off his cap, scratched his bald head and replaced the tattered headgear. 'THAT'S A BUGGER. GOOD PIG 'AN ALL. IS IT 'OPELESS?' He still gave tongue at the top of his voice despite his disappointment.

'Yes, I'm afraid it's pretty hopeless. They usually eat very little and just waste away. It would really be best to slaughter him.'

'NAY, AH DON'T LIKE THAT MUCH! AH ALLUS LIKE TO 'AVE A GO. ISN'T THERE SUMMAT WE CAN DO? WHERE THERE'S LIFE THERE'S 'OPE, THA KNAWS.'

I smiled. 'I suppose there's always some hope, Mr Hampson.'

'WELL THEN, LET'S GET ON. LET'S TRY!'

'All right.' I shrugged. 'He's not really in acute pain – more discomfort – so I suppose there's no harm in treating him. I'll leave you a course of powders.'

As I pushed my way from the pen I couldn't help noticing the superb sleek condition of the other pigs.

'My word,' I said. 'These pigs are in grand fettle. I've never seen a better lot. You must feed them well.'

It was a mistake. Enthusiasm added many decibels to his volume.

'*Aye!*' he bellowed. 'YOU'VE GOT TO GIVE STOCK A BIT O' GOOD STUFF TO MEK 'EM DO RIGHT!'

My head was still ringing when I reached the car and opened the boot. I handed over a packet of my faithful sulphonamide powders. They had done great things for me but I didn't expect much here.

It was strange that I should go straight from the chief shouter of the practice to the chief whisperer. Elijah Wentworth made all his communications *sotto voce*.

I found Mr Wentworth hosing down his cow byre and he turned and looked at me with his habitual serious expression. He was a tall thin man, very precise in his speech and ways, and though he was a hard-working farmer he didn't look like one. This impression was heightened by his clothes which were more suited to office work than his rough trade.

A fairly new trilby hat sat straight on his head as he came over to me. I was able to examine it thoroughly because he came so close that we were almost touching noses.

He took a quick look around him. 'Mr Herriot,' he whispered, 'I've got a real bad case.' He spoke always as though every pronouncement was of the utmost gravity and secrecy.

'Oh I'm sorry to hear that. What's the trouble?'

'Fine big bullock, Mr Herriot. Goin' down fast.' He moved in closer till he could murmur directly into my ear. 'I suspect TB.' He backed away, face drawn.

'That doesn't sound so good,' I said. 'Where is he?'

The farmer crooked a finger and I followed him into a loose box. The bullock was a Hereford Cross and should have weighed about ten hundredweight, but was gaunt and emaciated. I could understand Mr Wentworth's fears, but I was beginning to develop a clinical sense and it didn't look like TB to me.

'Is he coughing?' I asked.

'No, never coughs, but he's a bit skittered.'

I went over the animal carefully and there were a few things – the submaxillary oedema, the pot-bellied appearance, the pallor of the mucous membranes – which made diagnosis straightforward.

'I think he's got liver fluke, Mr Wentworth. I'll take a dung sample and have it examined for fluke eggs but I want to treat him right away.'

'Liver fluke? Where would he pick that up?'

'Usually from a wet pasture. Where has he been running lately?'

The farmer pointed through the door. 'Over yonder. I'll show you.'

I walked with him a few hundred yards and through a couple of gates into a wide flat field lying at the base of the fell. The squelchy feel of the turf and the scattered tufts of bog grass told the whole story.

'This is just the place for it,' I said. 'As you know, it's a parasite which infests the liver, but during its life cycle it has to pass through a snail and that snail can only live where there is water.'

He nodded slowly and solemnly several times then began to look around him and I knew he was going to say something. Again he came very close then scanned the horizon anxiously. In all directions the grassland stretched empty and bare for miles but he still seemed worried he might be overheard.

We were almost cheek to cheek as he breathed the words into my ear. 'Ah know who's to blame for this.'

'Really? Who is that?'

He made another swift check to ensure that nobody had sprung up through the ground then I felt his hot breath again. 'It's me landlord.'

'How do you mean?'

'Won't do anything for me.' He brought his face round and looked at me wide-eyed before taking up his old position by my ear. 'Been goin' to drain this field for years but done nowt.'

I moved back. 'Ah well, I can't help that, Mr Wentworth.

In any case there's other things you can do. You can kill the snails with copper sulphate – I'll tell you about that later – but in the meantime I want to dose your bullock.'

I had some hexachlorethane with me in the car and I mixed it in a bottle of water and administered it to the animal. Despite his bulk he offered no resistance as I held his lower jaw and poured the medicine down his throat.

'He's very weak, isn't he?' I said.

The farmer gave me a haggard look. 'He is that. I doubt he's a goner.'

'Oh don't give up hope, Mr Wentworth. I know he looks terrible but if it is fluke then the treatment will do a lot for him. Let me know how he goes on.'

It was about a month later, on a market day, and I was strolling among the stalls which packed the cobbles. In front of the entrance to the Drovers' Arms the usual press of farmers stood chatting among themselves, talking business with cattle dealers and corn merchants, while the shouts of the stallholders sounded over everything.

I was particularly fascinated by the man in charge of the sweet stall. He held up a paper bag and stuffed into it handfuls of assorted sweetmeats while he kept up a nonstop brazen-voiced commentary.

'Lovely peppermint drops! Delicious liquorice allsorts! How about some sugar candies! A couple o' bars o' chocolate! Let's 'ave some butterscotch an' all! Chuck in a beautiful slab o' Turkish Delight!' Then holding the bulging bag aloft in triumph ''ere! 'ere! Who'll give me a tanner for the lot?'

Amazing, I thought as I moved on. How did he do it? I was passing the door of the Drovers when a familiar voice hailed me.

'HEY! MR HERRIOT!' There was no mistaking Len Hampson. He hove in front of me, red-faced and cheerful. 'REMEMBER THAT PIG YE DOCTORED FOR ME?' He had clearly consumed a few market-day beers and his voice was louder than ever.

The packed mass of farmers pricked up their ears. There is nothing so intriguing as the ailments of another farmer's livestock.

'Yes, of course, Mr Hampson,' I replied.

'WELL 'E NEVER DID NO GOOD!' bawled Len.

I could see the farmers' faces lighting up. It is more interesting still when things go wrong.

'Really? Well I'm sorry.'

'NAW 'E DIDN'T. AH'VE NEVER SEEN A PIG GO DOWN AS FAST!'

'Is that so?'

'AYE, FLESH JUST MELTED OFF 'IM!'

'Oh, what a pity. But if you recall I rather expected . . .'

'WENT DOWN TO SKIN AND BONE 'E DID!' The great bellow rolled over the market place, drowning the puny cries of the stallholders. In fact the man with the sweets had suspended operations and was listening with as much interest as the others.

I looked around me uneasily. 'Well, Mr Hampson, I did warn you at the time . . .'

'LIKE A WALKIN' SKELETON 'E WERE! NEVER SEEN SUCH A OBJECK!'

I realized Len wasn't in the least complaining. He was just telling me, but for all that I wished he would stop.

'Well, thank you for letting me know,' I said. 'Now I really must be off . . .'

'AH DON'T KNOW WHAT THEM POWDERS WERE YOU GAVE 'IM.'

I cleared my throat. 'Actually they were . . .'

'THEY DID 'IM NO BLOODY GOOD ANY ROAD!'

'I see. Well as I say, I have to run . . .'

'AH GOT MALLOCK TO KNOCK 'IM ON T'HEAD LAST WEEK.'

'Oh dear . . .'

'FINISHED UP AS DOG MEAT, POOR BUGGER!'

'Quite . . . quite . . .'

'WELL, GOOD DAY TO YE, MR HERRIOT.' He turned and walked away, leaving a quivering silence behind him.

With an uncomfortable feeling that I was the centre of

attention I was about to retreat hastily when I felt a gentle hand on my arm. I turned and saw Elijah Wentworth.

'Mr Herriot,' he whispered. 'About that bullock.'

I stared at him, struck by the coincidence. The farmers stared, too, but expectantly.

'Yes, Mr Wentworth?'

'Well now, I'll tell you.' He came very near and breathed into my ear. 'It was like a miracle. He began to pick up straight away after you treated him.'

I stepped back. 'Oh marvellous! But speak up, will you, I can't quite hear you.' I looked around hopefully.

He came after me again and put his chin on my shoulder. 'Yes, I don't know what you gave 'im but it was wonderful stuff. I could hardly believe it. Every day I looked at 'im he had put on a bit more.'

'Great! But do speak a little louder,' I said eagerly.

'He's as fat as butter now.' The almost inaudible murmur wafted on my cheek. 'Ah'm sure he'll get top grade at the auction mart.'

I backed away again. 'Yes . . . yes . . . what was that you said?'

'I was sure he was dyin', Mr Herriot, but you saved him by your skill,' he said, but every word was pianissimo, sighed against my face.

The farmers had heard nothing and, their interest evaporating, they began to talk among themselves. Then as the man with the sweets started to fill his bags and shout again Mr Wentworth moved in and confided softly and secretly into my private ear.

'That was the most brilliant and marvellous cure I 'ave ever seen.'

twenty-five

It must be unusual to feel senile in one's twenties, but it was happening to me. There were a few men of my own age among my RAF friends but for the most part I was surrounded by eighteen- and nineteen-year-olds.

It seemed that the selection boards thought this the optimum age for training pilots, navigators and air gunners and I often wondered how we elderly gentlemen had managed to creep in.

These boys used to pull my leg. The fact that I was not merely married but a father put me in the dotage class, and the saddest part was that I really did feel old in their company. They were all having the most marvellous time; chasing the local girls, drinking, going to dances and parties, carried along on the frothy insouciance which a war engenders. And I often thought that if it had all happened a few years earlier I would have been doing the same.

But it was no good now. Most of me was still back in Darrowby. During the day there was enough pressure to keep my mind occupied but in the evenings when I was off the leash all I wanted to do were the simple things I had done with Helen; the long games of bezique by the fireside in our bed-sitter, tense battles on the push-ha'penny board; we even used to throw rings at hooks on a board on the wall. Kids' games after a hard slog round the practice, but even now as I look down the years I know I have never found a better way of living.

It was when we were lying in bed one night that Helen brought up the subject of Granville Bennett.

'Jim,' she murmured sleepily. 'Mr Bennett phoned again today. And his wife rang last week. They keep asking us to have a meal with them.'

'Yes . . . yes . . .' I didn't want to talk about anything at that moment. This was always a good time. The dying flames sent lights and shadows dancing across the ceiling, Oscar

Rabin's band was playing *Deep Purple* on the bedside radio Ewan Ross gave us for a wedding present and I had just pulled off an unexpected victory at push-ha'penny. Helen was a dab hand at that game, urging the coins expertly up the board with the ball of her thumb, her lips pushed forward in a pout of concentration. Of course she had a lifetime of experience behind her while I was just learning, and it was inevitable that I seldom won. But I had done it tonight and I felt good.

My wife nudged me with her knee. 'Jim, I can't understand you. You never seem to do anything about it. And yet you say you like him.'

'Oh, I do, he's a grand chap, one of the best.' Everybody liked Granville, but at the same time there were many strong men who dived down alleys at the sight of him. I didn't like to tell Helen that every time I came into contact with him I got my wings singed. I fully realized that he meant well, that the whole thing was a natural extension of his extreme generosity. But it didn't help.

'And you said his wife was very nice, too.'

'Zoe? Oh yes, she's lovely.' And she was, too, but thanks to her husband she had never seen me in any other role than a drunken hulk. My toes curled under the blankets. Zoe was beautiful, kind and intelligent – just the kind of woman you wanted to observe you staggering and hiccuping all over the place. In the darkness I could feel the hot blush of shame on my cheeks.

'Well then,' Helen continued, with the persistence that is part of even the sweetest women. 'Why don't we accept their invitation? I'd rather like to meet them – and it's a bit embarrassing when they keep phoning.'

I turned on my side. 'Okay, we'll go one of these days, I promise.'

But if it hadn't been for the little papilloma on Sam's lip I don't think we would ever have got there. I noticed the thing – a growth smaller than a pea – near the left commissure when I was giving our beagle an illicit chocolate biscuit. It was a typical benign tumour and on anybody else's dog I should have administered a quick local and whipped it off in a minute. But since it was Sam I turned pale and phoned Granville.

I have always been as soppy as any old lady over my pets and I suspect many of my colleagues are the same. I listened apprehensively to the buzz-buzz at the far end, then the big voice came on the line.

'Bennett here.'

'Hello, Granville, it's . . .'

'Jim!' The boom of delight was flattering. 'Where have you been hiding yourself, laddie?'

He didn't know how near he was to the truth. I told him about Sam.

'Doesn't sound much, old son, but I'll have a look at him with pleasure. Tell you what. We've been trying to get you over here for a meal – why not bring the little chap with you?'

'Well . . .' A whole evening in Granville's hands – it was a daunting prospect.

'Now don't mess about, Jim. You know, there's a wonderful Indian restaurant in Newcastle. Zoe and I would love to take you both out there. It's about time we met your wife, isn't it?'

'Yes . . . of course it is. . . . Indian restaurant, eh?'

'Yes, laddie. Superb curries – mild, medium or blast your bloody head off. Onion bhajis, bhuna lamb, gorgeous nan bread.'

My mind was working fast. 'Sounds marvellous, Granville.' It did seem fairly secure. He was most dangerous on his own territory and it would take forty-five minutes' driving each way to Newcastle. Then maybe an hour and a half in the restaurant. I should be reasonably safe for most of the evening. There was just the bit at his house before we left – that was the only worry.

It was uncanny how he seemed to read my thoughts. 'Before we leave, Jim, we'll have a little session in my garden.'

'Your garden?' It sounded strange in November.

'That's right, old lad.'

Ah well, maybe he was proud of his late chrysanthemums, and I couldn't see myself coming to much harm there. 'Well, fine, Granville. Maybe Wednesday night?'

'Lovely, lovely, lovely – can't wait to meet Helen.'

Wednesday was one of those bright frosty late autumn days which turn misty in the afternoon and by six o'clock the countryside was blanketed by one of the thickest fogs I had ever seen in Yorkshire.

Creeping along in our little car, my nose almost on the windscreen, I muttered against the glass.

'God's truth, Helen, we'll never get to Newcastle tonight! I know Granville's some driver but you can't see ten yards out there.'

Almost at walking pace we covered the twenty miles to the Bennett residence and it was with a feeling of relief that I saw the brightly lit doorway rising out of the mirk.

Granville, as vast and impressive as ever, was there in the hall with arms outspread. Bashfulness had never been one of his problems and he folded my wife in a bear-like embrace.

'Helen, my pet,' he said and kissed her fondly and lingeringly. He stopped to take a breath, regarded her for a moment with deep appreciation then kissed her again.

I shook hands decorously with Zoe and the two girls were introduced. They made quite a picture standing there. An attractive woman is a gift from heaven and it was a rare bonus to see two of them in close proximity. Helen very dark and blue-eyed, Zoe brown-haired with eyes of greyish-green, but both of them warm and smiling.

Zoe had her usual effect on me. That old feeling was welling up; the desire to look my best, in fact better than my best. I cast a furtive glance at the hall mirror. Immaculately suited, clean shirted, freshly shaven, I was sure I projected the desired image of the clean-limbed young veterinary surgeon, the newly married man of high principles and impeccable behaviour.

I breathed a silent prayer of thanks that at last she was seeing me stone cold sober and normal. Tonight I would expunge all her squalid memories of me from her mind.

'Zoe, my sweet,' carolled Granville. 'Take Helen into the garden while I see Jim's dog.'

I blinked. The garden in this fog. I just didn't get it, but I was too anxious about Sam to give the thing much thought. I opened the car door and the beagle trotted into the house.

My colleague greeted him with delight. 'Come inside, my little man.' Then he hollered at the top of his voice. 'Phoeble! Victoria! Yoo-hoo! Come and meet cousin Sam!'

The obese Staffordshire bull terrier waddled in, closely followed by the Yorkie, who bared her teeth in an ingratiating smile at all present.

After the dogs had met and exchanted pleasantries Granville lifted Sam into his arms.

'Is that what you mean, Jim? Is that what you're worried about?'

I nodded dumbly.

'Good God, I could take a deep breath and blow the damn thing off!' He looked at me incredulously and smiled. 'Jim, old lad, why are you so daft about your dog?'

'Why do you call Phoebe Phoebles?' I countered swiftly.

'Oh well . . .' He cleared his throat. 'I'll get my equipment. Hang on a minute.'

He disappeared and came back with a syringe and scissors. About half a cc was enough to numb the part, then he snipped off the papilloma, applied some stypic and put the beagle on the floor. The operation took about two minutes but even in that brief spell his unique dexterity was manifest.

'That'll be ten guineas, Mr Herriot,' he murmured, then gave a shout of laughter. 'Come on, let's get into the garden. Sam will be quite happy with my dogs.'

He led me out of the back door and we stumbled through the fog by a rockery and rose bushes. I was just wondering how on earth he expected to show me anything in this weather when we came up against a stone outhouse. He threw open the door and I stepped into a brightly lit, sparkling Aladdin's cave.

It was quite simply a fully fitted bar. At the far end a polished counter with beer handles and, behind, a long row of bottles of every imaginable liquor. A fire crackled in the hearth and hunting prints, cartoons and bright posters looked down from the walls. It was completely authentic.

Granville saw my astonished face and laughed. 'All right, eh, Jim? I thought it would be a nice idea to have my own little pub in the garden. Rather cosy, isn't it?'

'Yes . . . yes indeed . . . charming.'

'Good, good.' My colleague slipped behind the counter. 'Now what are you going to have?'

Helen and Zoe took sherry and I made a quick decision to stick to one fairly harmless drink.

'Gin and tonic, please, Granville.'

The girls received a normal measure of sherry but when the big man took my glass over to the gin bottle hanging on the wall his hand seemed to be overcome by an uncontrollable trembling. The bottle was upended with one of those little optic attachments you push up with the rim of the glass to give a single measure.

But as I say, as Granville inserted the neck of the bottle into the glass his whole arm jerked repeatedly as though he were going into a convulsion. It was obvious that the result would be about six gins instead of one and I was about to remonstrate when he took the glass away and topped it up quickly with tonic, ice and sliced lemon.

I looked at it apprehensively. 'Rather a big one, isn't it?'

'Not at all, laddie, nearly all tonic. Well, cheers, so nice to see you both.'

And it certainly was. They were generous, warm people and veterinary folk like ourselves. I felt a gush of gratitude for the friendliness they had always shown me and as I sipped my drink, which was chokingly strong, I felt as I had often done that these contacts were one of the brightest rewards of my job.

Granville held out his hand. 'Have another, laddie.'

'Well, hadn't we better be getting on our way? It's a terrible night – in fact I don't see us ever getting to Newcastle in this fog.'

'Nonsense, old son.' He took my glass, reached up to the

gin bottle and again was seized with a series of violent tremors of the forearm. 'No problem, Jim. Straight along the north road – half an hour or so – know it like the back of my hand.'

The four of us stood around the fire. The girls clearly had a lot to say to each other and Granville and I, like all vets, talked shop. It is wonderful how easy veterinary practice is in a warm room with good company and a dollop of alcohol in the stomach.

'One for the road, Jim,' my colleague said.

'No really, Granville, I've had enough,' I replied firmly. 'Let's be off.'

'Jim, Jim.' The familiar hurt look was creeping over his face. 'There's no rush. Look, we'll just have this last one while I tell you about this gorgeous restaurant.'

Once more he approached the gin bottle and this time the rigor lasted so long I wondered if he had some history of malaria.

Glass in hand he expounded. 'It's not just the curry, the cooking in general is exquisite.' He put his fingers to his lips and blew a reverent kiss into space. 'The flavours are unbelievable. All the spices of the orient, Jim.'

He went on at length and I wished he would stop because he was making me hungry. I had had a hard day round the farms and had eaten very little with the evening's feast in view, and as my colleague waved his hand around and drew word pictures of how they blended the rare herbs with the meat and fish, then served it on a bed of saffron rice, I was almost drooling.

I was relieved when I got through the third massive drink and Granville squeezed round to the front of the bar as if ready to go. We were on our way out when a man's bulk loomed in the doorway.

'Raymond!' cried Granville in delight. 'Come in, I've been wanting you to meet Jim Herriot. Jim, this is one of my neighbours – likes a bit of gardening, don't you Raymond?'

The man replied with a fat chuckle. 'Right, old boy! Splendid garden, this!' Granville seemed to know a lot of large, red-faced hearty men and this was one more.

My friend was behind the counter again. 'We must just have one with Raymond.'

I felt trapped as he again pressed my glass against the bottle and went into another paroxysm, but the girls didn't seem to mind. They were still deep in conversation and seemed unaware of the passage of time or the ravages of hunger.

Raymond was just leaving when Tubby Pinder dropped in. He was another enthusiastic horticulturist and I wasn't surprised to see that he was large, red-faced and hearty.

We had to have one with Tubby and I noticed with some alarm that after another palsied replenishment of my glass he had to replace the empty gin bottle with a fresh one. If the first one had been full then I had consumed nearly all of it.

I could hardly believe it when at last we were in the hall putting on our coats. Granville was almost purring with contentment.

'You two are going to love this place. It will be a joy to lead you through the menu.'

Outside the fog was thicker than ever. My colleague backed his enormous Bentley from the garage and began to usher us inside with great ceremony. He installed Helen and Zoe in the back, clucking solicitously over them, then he helped me into the passenger seat in front as though I were a disabled old man, tucking my coat in, adjusting the angle of the seat for maximum comfort, showing me how the cigar lighter worked, lighting up the glove compartment, enquiring which radio programme I desired.

At last he himself was in residence behind the wheel, massive and composed. Beyond the windscreen the fog parted for a second to show a steep, almost vertical grassy bank opposite the house, then it closed down like a dirty yellow curtain cutting off everything.

'Granville,' I said. 'We'll never get to Newcastle in this. It's over thirty miles.'

He turned and gave me a gentle smile. 'Absolutely no problem, laddie. We'll be there in half an hour, sampling that wonderful food. Tandoori chicken, all the spices of the orient, old son. Don't worry about a thing – I really know these roads. No chance of losing my way.'

He started the engine and drove confidently off, but unfortunately instead of taking the orthodox route along the road he proceeded straight up the grassy bank. He didn't seem to notice as the nose of the great car rose steadily higher, but when we had achieved an angle of forty-five degrees Zoe broke in gently from the back.

'Granville, dear, you're on the grass.'

My colleague looked round in some surprise. 'Not at all, my love. The road slopes a little here if you remember.' He kept his foot on the throttle.

I said nothing as my feet rose and my head went back. There was a point when the Bentley was almost perpendicular and I thought we were going over backwards, then I heard Zoe again.

'Granville, darling.' There was a hint of urgency in her tone. 'You're going up the bank.'

This time it seemed her husband was prepared to concede a little.

'Yes . . . yes, my pet,' he murmured as we hung there, all four of us gazing up at the fog-shrouded sky. 'Possibly I have strayed a little on to the verge.'

He took his foot off the brake and the car shot backwards at frightening speed into the darkness. We were brought up by a grinding crunch from the rear.

Zoe again: 'You've hit Mrs Thompson's wall, dear.'

'Have I, sweetheart? Ah, one moment. We'll soon be on our way.'

With undiminished aplomb he let in his clutch and we surged forward powerfully. But only for two seconds. From the gloom ahead there sounded a dull crash followed by a tinkling of glass and metal.

'Darling,' Zoe piped. 'That was the thirty miles an hour sign.'

'Was it really, my angel?' Granville rubbed his hand on the window. 'You know, Jim, the visibility isn't too good.'

He paused for a moment. 'Perhaps it would be a good idea if we postponed our visit till another time.'

He manoeuvred the big car back into the garage and we got out. We had covered, I should think, about five yards on our journey to Newcastle.

Back in the garden bar, Granville was soon in full cry again. And I was all for it because my earlier trepidation had vanished entirely. I was floating in a happy haze and I offered no resistance as my colleague jerked and twitched more samples from the gin bottle.

Suddenly he held up a hand. 'I'm sure we're all starving. Let's have some hot dogs!'

'Hot dogs?' I cried. 'Splendid idea!' It was a long call from all the spices of the orient but I was ready for anything.

'Zoe, sweet,' he said. 'We can use the big can of saveloy sausages if you would just heat it up.'

His wife left for the kitchen and Helen touched my arm.

'Jim,' she said. 'Saveloys . . . ?'

I knew what she meant. I have a pretty good digestion but there are certain things I can't eat. A single saveloy was enough to bring my entire metabolism to a halt, but at that moment it seemed a pettifogging detail.

'Oh don't worry, Helen,' I whispered, putting my arm round her. 'They won't hurt me.'

When Zoe came back with the food Granville was in his element, slicing the juicy smoked sausages lengthways, slapping mustard on them and enclosing them in rolls.

As I bit into the first one I thought I had never tasted anything so delicious. Chewing happily I found it difficult to comprehend my previous ridiculous prejudice.

'Ready for another, old son?' Granville held up a loaded roll.

'Sure! These are absolutely marvellous. Best hot dogs I've ever tasted!' I munched it down quickly and reached for a third.

I think it was when I had downed five of them that my friend prodded me in the ribs.

'Jim, lad,' he said between chews. 'We want a drop of beer to wash these down, don't you agree?'

I waved an arm extravagantly. 'Of course we do! Bloody gin's no good for this job!'

Granville pulled two pints of draught. Powerful delicious ale which flowed in a cooling wave over my inflamed mucous membranes, making me feel I had been waiting for it all my life. We each had three pints and another hot dog or two while waves of euphoria billowed around me.

The occasional anxious glance from Helen didn't worry me in the least. She was making signs that it was time to go home, but the very idea was unthinkable. I was having the time of my life, the world was a wonderful place and this little private pub was the finest corner of it.

Granville put down a half-eaten roll. 'Zoe, my precious, it would be nice to have something sweet to top this off. Why don't you bring out some of those little gooey things you made yesterday?'

She produced a plateful of very rich-looking cakelets. I do not have a sweet tooth and normally skip this part of the meal but I bit into one of Zoe's creations with relish. It was beautifully made and I could detect chocolate, marzipan, caramel and other things.

It was when I was eating the third that matters began to deteriorate. I found that my merry chatter had died and it was Granville doing all the talking, and as I listened to him owlishly I was surprised to see his face becoming two faces which floated apart and came together repeatedly. It was an astonishing phenomenon and it was happening with everything else in the room.

And I wasn't feeling so healthy now. That boundless vigour was no longer surging through my veins and I felt only a great weariness and a rising nausea.

I lost count of time around then. No doubt the conversation went on among the four of us but I can't remember any of it and my next recollection was of the party breaking up. Granville was helping Helen on with her coat and there was a general air of cheerful departure.

'Ready, Jim?' my friend said briskly.

I nodded and got slowly to my feet and as I swayed he put his arm round me and assisted me to the door. Outside, the fog had cleared and a bright pattern of stars overhung the village, but the clean cold air only made me feel worse and I stumbled through the darkness like a sleepwalker. When I reached the car a long griping spasm drove through me, reminding me horribly of the sausages, the gin and the rest. I groaned and leaned on the roof.

'Maybe you'd better drive, Helen,' my colleague said. He was about to open the door when, with a dreadful feeling of helplessness, I began to slide along the metal.

Granville caught my shoulders. 'He'd be better in the back,' he gasped and began to lug me on to the seat. 'Zoe, sweetheart, Helen, love, grab a leg each, will you? Fine, now I'll get round the other side and pull him in.'

He trotted round to the far side, opened the door and hauled at my shoulders.

'Down a bit your side, Helen, dear. Now to me a little. Up a trifle your side, Zoe, pet. Now back to you a bit. Lovely, lovely.'

Clearly he was happy at his work. He sounded like an expert furniture remover and through the mists I wondered bitterly how many inert forms he had stuffed into their cars after an evening with him.

Finally they got me in, half lying across the back seat. My face was pressed against the side window and from the outside it must have been a grotesque sight with the nose squashed sideways and a solitary dead-mackerel eye staring sightlessly into the night.

With an effort I managed to focus and saw Zoe looking down at me anxiously. She gave a tentative wave of goodbye but I could produce only a slight twitch of the cheek in reply.

Granville kissed Helen fondly then slammed the car door. Moving back, he peered in at me and brandished his arms.

'See you soon, I hope, Jim. It's been a lovely evening!' His big face was wreathed in a happy smile and as we drove away my final impression was that he was thoroughly satisfied.

twenty-six

Being away from Darrowby and living a different life I was able to stand back and assess certain things objectively. I asked myself many questions. Why, for instance, was my partnership with Siegfried so successful?

Even now, as we still jog along happily after thirty-five years, I wonder about it. I know I liked him instinctively when I first saw him in the garden at Skeldale House on that very first afternoon, but I feel there is another reason why we get on together.

Maybe it is because we are opposites. Siegfried's restless energy impels him constantly to try to alter things while I abhor change of any kind. A lot of people would call him brilliant, while not even my best friends would apply that description to me. His mind relentlessly churns out ideas of all grades – excellent, doubtful and very strange indeed. I, on the other hand, rarely have an idea of any sort. He likes hunting, shooting and fishing; I prefer football, cricket and tennis. I could go on and on – we are even opposite physical types – and yet, as I say, we get along.

This of course doesn't mean that we have never had our differences. Over the years there have been minor clashes on various points.

One, I recall, was over the plastic calcium injectors. They were something new so Siegfried liked them, and by the same token I regarded them with deep suspicion.

My doubts were nourished by my difficulties with them. Their early troubles have now been ironed out but at the beginning I found the things so temperamental that I abandoned them.

My colleague pulled me up about it when he saw me washing out my flutter valve by running the surgery tap through it.

'For God's sake, James, you're not still using that old thing, are you?'

'Yes, I'm afraid I am.'

'But haven't you tried the new plastics?'

'I have.'

'Well . . . ?'

'Can't get away with them, Siegfried.'

'Can't . . . what on earth do you mean?'

I trickled the last drop of water through the tube, rolled it small and slipped it into its case. 'Well, the last time I used one the calcium squirted all over the place. And it's messy, sticky stuff. I had great white streaks down my coat.'

'But James!' He laughed incredulously. 'That's crazy! They're childishly simple to use. I haven't had the slightest trouble.'

'I believe you,' I said. 'But you know me. I haven't got a mechanical mind.'

'For heaven's sake, you don't need a mechanical mind. They're foolproof.'

'Not to me, they aren't. I've had enough of them.'

My colleague put his hand on my shoulder and his patient look began to creep across his face. 'James, James, you must persevere.' He raised a finger. 'There is another point at issue here, you know.'

'What's that?'

'The matter of asepsis. How do you know that length of rubber you have there is clean?'

'Well, I wash it through after use, I use a boiled needle, and . . .'

'But don't you see, my boy, you're only trying to achieve what already exists in the plastic pack. Each one is self-contained and sterilized.'

'Oh I know all about that, but what's the good of it if I can't get the stuff into the cow?' I said querulously.

'Oh piffle, James!' Siegfried assumed a grave expression. 'It only needs a little application on your part, and I must stress that you are behaving in a reactionary manner by being stubborn. I put it to you seriously that we have to move with the times and every time you use that antiquated outfit of yours it is a retrograde step.'

We stood, as we often did, eyeball to eyeball, in mutual

disagreement till he smiled suddenly. 'Look, you're going out now, aren't you, to see that milk-fever cow I treated at John Tillot's. I understand it's not up yet.'

'That's right.'

'Well, as a favour to me, will you give one of the new packs a try?'

I thought for a moment. 'All right, Siegfried, I'll have one more go.'

When I reached the farm I found the cow comfortably ensconced in a field, in the middle of a rolling yellow ocean of buttercups.

'She's had a few tries to get on 'er feet,' the farmer said. 'But she can't quite make it.'

'Probably just wants another shot.' I went to my car which I had driven, rocking and bumping, over the rig and furrow of the field, and took one of the plastic packs from the boot.

Mr Tillot raised his eyebrows when he saw me coming back. 'Is that one o' them new things?'

'Yes, it is, Mr Tillot, the very latest invention. All completely sterilized.'

'Ah don't care what it is, ah don't like it!'

'You don't?'

'Naw!'

'Well . . . why not?'

'Ah'll tell ye. Mr Farnon used one this mornin'. Some of the stuff went in me eye, some went in 'is ear 'ole and the rest went down 'is trousers. Ah don't think t'bloody cow got any!'

There was another time Siegfried had to take me to task. An old-age pensioner was leading a small mongrel dog along the passage on the end of a piece of string. I patted the consulting room table.

'Put him up here, will you?' I said.

The old man bent over slowly, groaning and puffing.

'Wait a minute.' I tapped his shoulder. 'Let me do it.' I hoisted the little animal on to the smooth surface.

'Thank ye, sir.' The man straightened up and rubbed his back and leg. 'I 'ave arthritis bad and I'm not much good at liftin'. My name's Bailey and I live at t'council houses.'

'Right, Mr Bailey, what's the trouble?'

'It's this cough. He's allus at it. And 'e kind of retches at t'end of it.'

'I see. How old is he?'

'He were ten last month.'

'Yes . . .' I took the temperature and carefully auscultated the chest. As I moved the stethoscope over the ribs Siegfried came in and began to rummage in the cupboard.

'It's a chronic bronchitis, Mr Bailey,' I said. 'Many older dogs suffer from it just like old folks.'

He laughed. 'Aye, ah'm a bit wheezy meself sometimes.'

'That's right, but you're not so bad, really, are you?'

'Naw, naw.'

'Well neither is your little dog. I'm going to give him an injection and a course of tablets and it will help him quite a bit. I'm afraid he'll never quite get rid of this cough, but bring him in again if it gets very bad.'

He nodded vigorously. 'Very good, sir. Thank ye kindly, sir.'

As Siegfried banged about in the cupboard I gave the injection and counted out twenty of the new M&B 693 tablets.

The old man gazed at them with interest then put them in his pocket. 'Now what do ah owe ye, Mr Herriot?'

I looked at the ragged tie knotted carefully over the frayed shirt collar, at the threadbare antiquity of the jacket. His trouser knees had been darned but on one side I caught a pink glimpse of the flesh through the material.

'No, that's all right, Mr Bailey. Just see how he goes on.'

'Eh?'

'There's no charge.'

'But . . .'

'Now don't worry about it – it's nothing, really. Just see he gets his tablets regularly.'

'I will, sir, and it's very kind of you. I never expected . . .'

'I know you didn't, Mr Bailey. Goodbye for now and bring him back if he's not a lot better in a few days.'

The sound of the old man's footsteps had hardly died away when Siegfried emerged from the cupboard. He brandished a pair of horse tooth forceps in my face. 'God, I've been ages hunting these down. I'm sure you deliberately hide things from me, James.'

I smiled but made no reply and as I was replacing my syringe on the trolley my colleague spoke again.

'James, I don't like to mention this, but aren't you rather rash, doing work for nothing?'

I looked at him in surprise. 'He was an old-age pensioner. Pretty hard up I should think.'

'Maybe so, but really, you know, you just cannot give your services free.'

'Oh but surely occasionally, Siegfried – in a case like this . . .'

'No, James, not even occasionally. It's just not practical.'

'But I've seen you do it – time and time again!'

'Me?' His eyes widened in astonishment. 'Never! I'm too aware of the harsh realities of life for that. Everything has become so frightfully expensive. For instance, weren't those M&B 693 tablets you were dishing out? Heaven help us, do you know those things are threepence each? It's no good – you must never work without charging.'

'But dammit, you're always doing it!' I burst out. 'Only last week there was that . . .'

Siegfried held up a restraining hand. 'Please, James, please. You imagine things, that's your trouble.'

I must have given him one of my most exasperated stares because he reached out and patted my shoulder.

'Believe me, my boy, I do understand. You acted from the highest possible motives and I have often been tempted to do the same. But you must be firm. These are hard times and one must be hard to survive. So remember in future – no more Robin Hood stuff, we can't afford it.'

I nodded and went on my way somewhat bemusedly, but I soon forgot the incident and would have thought no more about it had I not seen Mr Bailey about a week later.

His dog was once more on the consulting room table and

Siegfried was giving it an injection. I didn't want to interfere so I went back along the passage to the front office and sat down to write in the day book. It was a summer afternoon, the window was open and through a parting in the curtain I could see the front steps.

As I wrote I heard Siegfried and the old man passing on their way to the front door. They stopped on the steps. The little dog, still on the end of its string, looked much as it did before.

'All right, Mr Bailey,' my colleague said. 'I can only tell you the same as Mr Herriot. I'm afraid he's got that cough for life, but when it gets bad you must come and see us.'

'Very good, sir,' the old man put his hand in his pocket. 'And what is the charge, please?'

'The charge, oh yes . . . the charge . . .' Siegfried cleared his throat a few times but seemed unable to articulate. He kept looking from the mongrel dog to the old man's tattered clothing and back again. Then he glanced furtively into the house and spoke in a hoarse whisper.

'It's nothing, Mr Bailey.'

'But Mr Farnon, I can't let ye . . .'

'Shh! Shh!' Siegfried waved a hand agitatedly in the old man's face. 'Not a word now! I don't want to hear any more about it.'

Having silenced Mr Bailey he produced a large bag.

'There's about a hundred M&B tablets in here,' he said, throwing an anxious glance over his shoulder. 'He's going to keep needing them, so I've given you a good supply.'

I could see my colleague had spotted the hole in the trouser knee because he gazed down at it for a long time before putting his hand in his jacket pocket.

'Hang on a minute.' He extracted a handful of assorted chattels. A few coins fell and rolled down the steps as he prodded in his palm among scissors, thermometers, pieces of string, bottle openers. Finally his search was rewarded and he pulled out a bank note.

'Here's a quid,' he whispered and again nervously shushed the man's attempts to speak.

Mr Bailey, realizing the futility of argument, pocketed the money.

'Well, thank ye, Mr Farnon. Ah'll take t'missus to Scarborough wi' that.'

'Good lad, good lad,' muttered Siegfried, still looking around him guiltily. 'Now off you go.'

The old man solemnly raised his cap and began to shuffle painfully down the street.

'Hey, hold on, there,' my colleague called after him. 'What's the matter? You're not going very well.'

'It's this dang arthritis. Ah go a long way in a long time.'

'And you've got to walk all the way to the council houses?' Siegfried rubbed his chin irresolutely. 'It's a fair step.' He took a last wary peep down the passage then beckoned with his hand.

'Look, my car's right here,' he whispered. 'Nip in and I'll run you home.'

Some of our disagreements were sharp and short.

I was sitting at the lunch table, rubbing and flexing my elbow. Siegfried, carving enthusiastically at a joint of roast mutton, looked up from his work.

'What's the trouble, James – rheumatism?'

'No, a cow belted me with her horn this morning. Right on the funny bone.'

'Oh, bad luck. Were you trying to get hold of her nose?'

'No, giving her an injection.'

My colleague, transporting a slice of mutton to my plate, paused in mid-air. 'Injecting her? Up there?'

'Yes, in the neck.'

'Is that where you do it?'

'Yes, always have done. Why?'

'Because if I may say so, it's rather a daft place. I always use the rump.'

'Is that so?' I helped myself to mashed potatoes. 'And what's wrong with the neck?'

'Well, you've illustrated it yourself, haven't you? It's too damn near the horns for a start.'

'Okay, well the rump is too damn near the hind feet.'

'Oh, come now, James, you know very well a cow very seldom kicks after a rump injection.'

'Maybe so, but once is enough.'

'And once is enough with a bloody horn, isn't it?'

I made no reply, Siegfried plied the gravy boat over both our plates and we started to eat. But he had hardly swallowed the first mouthful when he returned to the attack.

'Another thing, the rump is so handy. Your way you have to squeeze up between the cows.'

'Well, so what?'

'Simply that you get your ribs squashed and your toes stood on, that's all.'

'All right.' I spooned some green beans from the tureen. 'But your way you stand an excellent chance of receiving a faceful of cow shit.'

'Oh rubbish, James, you're just making excuses!' He hacked violently at his mutton.

'Not at all,' I said. 'It's what I believe. And anyway, you haven't made out a case against the neck.'

'Made out a case? I haven't started yet. I could go on indefinitely. For instance, the neck is more painful.'

'The rump is more subject to contamination,' I countered.

'The neck is often thinly muscled,' snapped Siegfried. 'You haven't got a nice pad there to stick your needle into.'

'No, and you haven't got a tail either,' I growled.

'Tail? What the hell are you talking about?'

'I'm talking about the bloody tail! It's all right if you have somebody holding it but otherwise it's a menace, lashing about.'

Siegfried gave a few rapid chews and swallowed quickly. 'Lashing about? What in God's name has that got to do with it?'

'Quite a lot,' I replied. 'I don't like a whack across the face from a shitty tail, even if you do.'

There was a heavy-breathing lull then my colleague spoke in an ominously quiet voice. 'Anything else about the tail?'

'Yes, there is. Some cows can whip a syringe out of your

hand with their tail. The other day one caught my big fifty cc and smashed it against a wall. Broken glass everywhere.'

Siegfried flushed slightly and put down his knife and fork. 'James, I don't like to speak to you in these terms, but I am bound to tell you that you are talking the most unmitigated balls, bullshit and poppycock.'

I gave him a sullen glare. 'That's your opinion, is it?'

'It is indeed, James.'

'Right.'

'Right.'

'Okay.'

'Very well.'

We continued our meal in silence.

But over the next few days my mind kept returning to the conversation. Siegfried has always had a persuasive way with him and the thought kept recurring that there might be a lot in what he said.

It was a week later that I paused, syringe in hand, before pushing between two cows. The animals, divining my intent as they usually did, swung their craggy hind ends together and blocked my way. Yes, by God, Siegfried had a point. Why should I fight my way in there when the other end was ready and waiting?

I came to a decision. 'Hold the tail, please,' I said to the farmer and pushed my needle into the rump.

The cow never moved and as I completed the injection and pulled the needle out I was conscious of a faint sense of shame. That lovely pad of gluteal muscle, the easy availability of the site – my colleague had been dead right and I had been a pig-headed fool. I knew what to do in future.

The farmer laughed as he stepped back across the dung channel. 'It's a funny thing how you fellers all have your different ways.'

'What do you mean?'

'Well, Mr Farnon was 'ere yesterday, injecting that cow over there.'

'He was?' A sudden light flashed in my mind. Could it be

that Siegfried was not the only convincing talker in our practice . . . ? 'What about it?'

' Just that 'e had a different system from you. He injected into the neck.'

twenty-seven

I leaned on the handle of my spade, wiped away the sweat which had begun to run into my eyes and gazed around me at the hundreds of men scattered over the dusty green.

We were still on our toughening course. At least that's what they told us it was. I had a private suspicion that they just didn't know what to do with all the aircrews under training and that somebody had devised this method of getting us out of the way.

Anyway, we were building a reservoir near a charming little Shropshire town and a whole village of tents had sprung up to house us. Nobody was quite sure about the reservoir but we were supposed to be building something. They issued us with denim suits and pick-axes and spades and for hour after hour we pecked desultorily at a rocky hillside.

But, hot as I was, I couldn't help thinking that things could be a lot worse. The weather was wonderful and it was a treat to be in the open all day. I looked down the slope and away across the sweetly rolling countryside to where low hills rose in the blue distance; it was a gentler landscape than the stark fells and moors I had left behind in Yorkshire, but infinitely soothing.

And the roofs of the town showing above the trees held a rich promise. During the hours under the fierce sun, with the rock dust caking round our lips, we built up a gargantuan thirst which we nurtured carefully till the evening when we were allowed out of camp.

There, in cool taverns in the company of country folk, we

slaked it with pints of glorious rough cider. I don't suppose you would find any there now. It is mostly factory-made cider which is drunk in the South of England these days, but many of the pubs used to have their own presses where they squeezed the juice from the local apples.

To me, there was something disturbing about sleeping in a tent. Each morning when I awoke with the early sun beating on the thin walls it was as if I were back in the hills above the Firth of Clyde long before the war was dreamed of. There was something very evocative about the tent smell of hot canvas and rubber groundsheet and crushed grass and the flies buzzing in a little cloud at the top of the pole. I was jerked back in an instant to Rosneath and when I opened my eyes I half expected to find Alex Taylor and Eddie Hutchinson, the friends of my boyhood, lying there in their sleeping bags.

The three of us went camping at Rosneath every weekend from Easter to October, leaving the smoke and dirt of Glasgow behind us; and here in Shropshire, in the uncanny tent smell, when I closed my eyes I could see the little pinewood behind the tent and the green hillside running down to the burn and, far below, the long blue mirror of the Gareloch glinting under the great mountains of Argyll. They have desecrated Rosneath and the Gareloch now, but to me, as a boy, it was a fairyland which led me into the full wonder and beauty of the world.

It was strange that I should dwell on that period when I was in my teens because Alex was in the Middle East, Eddie was in Burma and I was in another tent with a lot of different young men. And it was as though the time between had been rubbed away and Darrowby and Helen and all my struggles in veterinary practice had never happened. Yet those years in Darrowby had been the most important of my life. I used to sit up and shake myself, wondering at how my thoughts had been mixed up by the war.

But as I say, I quite enjoyed Shropshire. The only snag was that reservoir, or whatever it was that we were hacking out of the face of the hill. I could never get really involved with it.

So that I pricked up my ears when our Flight Sergeant made an announcement one morning.

'Some of the local farmers want help with their harvest,' he called out at the early parade. 'Are there any volunteers?'

My hand was the first up and after a few moments' hesitation others followed, but none of my particular friends volunteered for the job. When everything had been sorted out I found I had been allotted to a farmer Edwards with three other airmen who were from a different flight and strangers to me.

Mr Edwards arrived the following day and packed the four of us into a typical big old-fashioned farmer's car. I sat in the front with him while the three others filled the back. He asked our names but nothing else, as though he felt that our station in civil life was none of his concern. He was about thirty-five with jet black hair above a sunburnt face in which his white teeth and clear blue eyes shone startlingly.

He looked us over with a good-humoured grin as we rolled into his farmyard.

'Well, here we are, lads,' he said. 'This is where we're going to put you through it.'

But I hardly heard him. I was looking around me at the scene which had been part of my life a few months ago. The cobbled yard, the rows of doors leading to cow byre, barn, pigsties and loose boxes. An old man was mucking out the byre and as the rich bovine smell drifted across, one of my companions wrinkled his nose. But I inhaled it like perfume.

The farmer led us all into the fields where a reaper and binder was at work, leaving the sheaves of corn lying in long golden swathes.

'Any of you ever done any stooking?' he asked.

We shook our heads dumbly.

'Never mind, you'll soon learn. You come with me, Jim.'

We spaced ourselves out in the big field, each of my colleagues with an old man while Mr Edwards took charge of me. It didn't take me long to realize that I had got the tough section.

The farmer grabbed a sheaf in each hand, tucked them

230

under his arms, walked a few steps and planted them on end, resting against each other. I did the same till there were eight sheaves making up a stook. He showed me how to dig the stalks into the ground so that they stood upright and sometimes he gave a nudge with his knee to keep them in the right alignment.

I did my best but often my sheaves would fall over and I had to dart back and replace them. And I noticed with some alarm that Mr Edwards was going about twice as fast as the three old men. We had nearly finished the row while they were barely half way along, and my aching arms and back told me I was in for a testing time.

We went on like that for about two hours; bending, lifting, bending, lifting and shuffling forward without an instant's respite. One of the strongest impressions I had gained when I first came into country practice was that farming was the hardest way of all of making a living, and now I was finding out for myself. I was about ready to throw myself down on the stubble when Mrs Edwards came over the field with her young son and daughter. They carried baskets with the ingredients for our ten o'clock break; crusty apple tart and jugs of cider.

The farmer watched me quizzically as I sank gratefully down and began to drink like a parched traveller in the desert. The cider, from his own press, was superb, and I closed my eyes as I swallowed. The right thing, it seemed to me, would be to lie here in the sunshine for the rest of the day with about a gallon of this exquisite brew by my side, but Mr Edwards had other ideas. I was still chewing at the solid crust when he grasped a fresh pair of sheaves.

'Right, lad, must get on,' he grunted, and I was back on the treadmill.

With a pause at lunchtime for bread, cheese and more cider we went on at breakneck speed all day. I have always been grateful to the RAF for what they did for my physical well-being. When I was called up there was no doubt I was going slightly to seed under Helen's beneficent regime. Too much good cooking and the discovery of the charms of an armchair; I was getting fat. But the RAF changed all that and I don't think I have ever slipped back.

After the six months at Scarborough I am certain I didn't carry a surplus pound. Marching, drilling, PT, running – I could trot five miles along the beach and cliffs without trouble. When I arrived in Shropshire I was really fit. But I wasn't as fit as Mr Edwards.

He was a compact bundle of power. Not very big but with the wiry durability I remembered in the Yorkshire farmers. He seemed tireless, hardly breaking sweat as he moved along the rows, corded brown arms bulging from the sleeves of a faded collarless shirt, slightly bowed legs stumping effortlessly.

The sensible thing would have been to tell him straight that I couldn't go at his pace, but some demon of pride impelled me to keep up with him. I am quite sure he didn't mean to rub it in. Like any other farmer he had a job to do and was anxious to get on with it. At the lunch break he looked at me with some commiseration as I stood there, shirt sticking to my back, mouth hanging open, ribs heaving.

'You're doin' fine, Jim,' he said, then, as if noticing my distress for the first time, he shifted his feet awkwardly. 'I know you city lads ain't used to this kind of work and . . . well . . . it's not a question of strength, it's just knowin' how to do it.'

When we drove back to camp that night I could hear my companions groaning in the back of the car. They, too, had suffered, but not as badly as me.

After a few days I did begin to get the knack of the thing and though it still tested me to the utmost I was never on the border of collapse again.

Mr Edwards noticed the improvement and slapped me playfully on the shoulder. 'What did I tell you? It's just knowin' how to do it!'

But a new purgatory awaited me when we started to load the corn on to the stack. Forking the sheaves up on to the cart, roping them there then throwing them again, higher and higher as the stack grew in size. I realized with a jolt that stooking had been easy.

Mrs Edwards joined in this part. She stood on the top of

the stack with her husband, expertly turning the sheaves towards him while he arranged them as they should be. I had the unskilled job way below, toiling as never before, back breaking, the handle of the fork blistering my palms.

I just couldn't go fast enough and Mr Edwards had to hop down to help me, grasping a fork and hurling the sheaves up with easy flicks of the wrist.

He looked at me as before and spoke the encouraging words. 'You're comin' along grand, Jim. It's just knowin' how to do it.'

But there were many compensations. The biggest was being among farming folk again. Mrs Edwards in her undemonstrative way was obviously anxious to show hospitality to these four rather bewildered city boys far from home, and set us down to a splendid meal every evening. She was dark like her husband, with large eyes which joined in her quick smile and a figure which managed to be thin and shapely at the same time. She hadn't much chance to get fat because she never stopped working. When she wasn't outside throwing the corn around like any man she was cooking and baking, looking after her children and scouring her great barn of a farmhouse.

Those evening meals were something to look forward to and remember. Steaming rabbit pies with fresh green beans and potatoes from the garden. Bilberry tarts and apple crumble and a massive jug of thick cream to pour ad lib. Home-baked bread and farm cheese.

The four of us revelled in the change from the RAF fare. It was said the aircrews got the best food in the services and I believed it, but after a while it all began to taste the same. Maybe it was the bulk cooking but it palled in time.

Sitting at the farm table, looking at Mrs Edwards serving us, at her husband eating stolidly and at the two children, a girl of ten whose dark eyes showed promise of her mother's attractiveness and a sturdy, brown-limbed boy of eight, the thought recurred; they were good stock.

The clever economists who tell us that we don't need British agriculture and that our farms should be turned into national parks seem to ignore the rather obvious snag that an unfriendly country could starve us into submission in a week. But to me a greater tragedy still would be the loss of a whole community of people like the Edwards.

It was late one afternoon and I was feeling more of a weakling than ever, with Mr Edwards throwing the sheaves around as though they were weightless while I groaned and strained. The farmer was called away to attend to a calving cow and as he hopped blithely from the stack he patted my shoulder as I leaned on my fork.

'Never mind, Jim,' he laughed. 'It's just knowin' how to do it.'

An hour later we were going into the kitchen for our meal when Mrs Edwards said, 'My husband's still on with that cow. He must be having difficulty with her.'

I hesitated in the doorway. 'Do you mind if I go and see how he's getting on?'

She smiled. 'All right, if you like. I'll keep your food warm for you.'

I crossed the yard and went into the byre. One of the old men was holding the tail of a big Red Poll and puffing his pipe placidly. Mr Edwards, stripped to the waist, had his arm in the cow up to the shoulder. But it was a different Mr Edwards. His back and chest glistened and droplets of sweat ran down his nose and dripped steadily from the end. His mouth gaped and he panted as he fought his private battle somewhere inside.

He turned glazed eyes in my direction. At first he didn't appear to see me in his absorption, then recognition dawned.

''Ullo, Jim,' he muttered breathlessly. 'I've got a right job on 'ere.'

'Sorry to hear that. What's the trouble?'

He began to reply then screwed up his face. 'Aaah! The old bitch! She's squeezin' the life out of me arm again! She'll break it afore she's finished!' He paused, head hanging down, to recover, then he looked up at me. 'The calf's laid wrong, Jim. There's just a tail comin' into the passage and I can't get the hind legs round.'

A breech. My favourite presentation but one which always defeated farmers. I couldn't blame them really because they

234

had never had the opportunity to read Franz Benesch's classical work on *Veterinary Obstetrics* which explains the mechanics of parturition so lucidly. One phrase has always stuck in my mind: 'The necessity for simultaneous application of antagonistic forces'.

Benesch points out that in order to correct many malpresentations it is necessary to apply traction and repulsion at the same time, and to do that with one hand in a straining cow is impossible.

As though to endorse my thoughts Mr Edwards burst out once more. 'Dang it, I've missed it again! I keep pushin' the hock away then grabbin' for the foot but the old bitch just shoves it all back at me. I've been doin' this for an hour now and I'm about knackered.'

I never thought I would hear such words from this tough little man, but there was no doubt he had suffered. The cow was a massive animal with a back like a dining table and she was heaving the farmer back effortlessly every time she strained. We didn't see many Red Polls in Yorkshire but the ones I had met were self-willed and strong as elephants; the idea of pushing against one for an hour made me quail.

Mr Edwards pulled his arm out and stood for a moment leaning against the hair rump. The animal was quite unperturbed by the interference of this puny human but the farmer was a picture of exhaustion. He worked his dangling fingers gingerly then looked up at me.

'By God!' he grunted. 'She's given me some stick. I've got hardly any feelin' left in this arm.'

He didn't have to tell me. I had known that sensation many a time. Even Benesch in the midst of his coldly scientific 'repositions', 'retropulsions', 'malpositions' and 'counteracting pressures' so far unbends as to state that 'Great demands are made upon the strength of the operator'. Mr Edwards would agree with him.

The farmer took a long shuddering breath and moved over to the bucket of hot water on the floor. He washed his arms then turned back to the cow with something like dread on his face.

'Look,' I said. 'Please let me help you.'

He gave a pallid smile. 'Thanks, Jim, but there's nuthin' you can do. Those legs have got to come round.'

'That's what I mean. I can do it.'

'What . . .?'

'With a bit of help from you. Have you got a piece of binder twine handy?'

'Aye, we've got yards of it, lad, but I'm tellin' you you need experience for this job. You know nuthin' about . . .'

He stopped because I was already pulling my shirt over my head. He was too tired to argue in any case.

Hanging the shirt on a nail on the wall, bending over the bucket and soaping my arms with the scent of the antiseptic coming up to me brought a rush of memories which was almost overwhelming. I held out my hand and Mr Edwards wordlessly passed me a length of twine.

I soaked it in the water, then quickly tied a slip knot at one end and inserted my hand into the cow. Ah yes, there was the tail, so familiar, hanging between the calf's pelvic bones. Oh, I did love a breach, and I ran my hand with almost voluptuous satisfaction along the hair of the limb till I reached the tiny foot. It was a moment's work to push the loop over the fetlock and tighten it while I passed the free end between the digits of the cloven foot.

'Hold that,' I said to the farmer, 'and pull it steadily when I tell you.'

I put my hand on the hock and began to push it away from me into the uterus.

'Now pull,' I said. 'But carefully. Don't jerk.'

Like a man in a dream he did as I said and within seconds the foot popped out of the vulva.

'Hell!' said Mr Edwards.

'Now for the other one,' I murmured as I removed the loop.

I repeated the procedure, the farmer, slightly pop-eyed, pulling on the twine. The second little hoof, yellow and moist, joined its fellow on the outside almost immediately.

'Bloody hell!' said Mr Edwards.

'Right,' I said. 'Grab a leg and we'll have him out in a couple of ticks.'

We each took a hold and leaned back, but the big cow did the job for us, giving a great heave which deposited the calf wet and wriggling into my arms. I staggered back and dropped with it on to the straw.

'Grand bull calf, Mr Edwards,' I said. 'Better give him a rub down.'

The farmer shot me a disbelieving glance then twisted some hay into a wisp and began to dry off the little creature.

'If you ever get stuck with a breech presentation again,' I said, 'I'll show you what you ought to do. You have to push and pull at the same time and that's where the twine comes in. As you repel the hock with your hand somebody else pulls the foot round, but you'll notice I have the twine between the calf's cleats and that's important. That way it lifts the sharp little foot up and prevents injury to the vaginal wall.'

The farmer nodded dumbly and went on with his rubbing. When he had finished he looked up at me in bewilderment and his lips moved soundlessly a few times before he spoke.

'What the . . . how . . . how the heck do you know all that?'

I told him.

There was a long pause then he exploded.

'You young bugger! You kept that dark, didn't you?'

'Well . . . you never asked me.'

He scratched his head. 'Well, I don't want to be nosey with you lads that helps me. Some folks don't like it . . .' His voice trailed away.

We dried our arms and donned our shirts in silence. Before leaving he looked over at the calf, already making strenuous efforts to rise as its mother licked it.

'He's a lively little beggar,' he said. 'And we might have lost 'im. I'm right grateful to you.' He put an arm round my shoulders. 'Anyway, come on, Mister Veterinary Surgeon, and we'll 'ave some supper.'

Half way across the yard he stopped and regarded me ruefully. 'You know, I must have looked proper daft to you, fumblin' away inside there for an hour and damn near killin' myself, then you step up and do it in a couple of minutes. I feel as weak as a girl.'

'Not in the least, Mr Edwards,' I replied. 'It's . . .' I hesitated a moment. 'It's not a question of strength, it's just knowing how to do it.'

He nodded, then became very still and the seconds stretched out as he stared at me. Suddenly his teeth shone as the brown face broke into an ever-widening grin which developed into a great shout of laughter.

He was still laughing helplessly when we reached the house and as I opened the kitchen door he leaned against the wall and wiped his eyes.

'You young divil!' he said. 'You really got a bit o' your own back there, didn't you?'

twenty-eight

At last we were on our way to Flying School. It was at Windsor and that didn't seem far on the map, but it was a typical war-time journey of endless stops and changes and interminable waits. It went on all through the night and we took our sleep in snatches. I stole an hour's fitful slumber on the waiting-room table at a tiny nameless station and despite my hard pillowless bed I drifted deliciously back to Darrowby.

I was bumping along the rutted track to Nether Lees Farm, hanging on to the jerking wheel. I could see the house below me, its faded red tiles showing above the sheltering trees, and behind the buildings the scrubby hillside rose to the moor.

Up there the trees were stunted and sparse and dotted widely over the steep flanks. Higher still there was only scree and cliff and right at the top, beckoning in the sunshine, I saw the beginning of the moor – smooth, unbroken and bare.

A scar on the broad sweep of green showed where long ago they quarried the stones to build the massive farmhouses and the enduring walls which have stood against the unrelenting climate for hundreds of years. Those houses and those endlessly marching walls would still be there when I was gone and forgotten.

Helen was with me in the car. I loved it when she came with me on my rounds, and after the visit to the farm we climbed up the fell-side, panting through the scent of the warm bracken, feeling the old excitement as we neared the summit.

Then we were on the top, facing into the wide free moorland and the clean Yorkshire wind and the cloud shadows racing over the greens and browns. Helen's hand was warm in mine as we wandered among the heather through green islets nibbled to a velvet sward by the sheep. She raised a finger as a curlew's lonely cry sounded across the wild tapestry and the wonder in her eyes shone through the dark flurry of hair blowing across her face.

The gentle shaking at my shoulder pulled me back to wakefulness, to the hiss of steam and the clatter of boots. The table top was hard against my hip and my neck was stiff where it had rested on my pack.

'Train's in, Jim.' An airman was looking down at me. 'I hated to wake you – you were smiling.'

Two hours later, sweaty, unshaven, half asleep, laden with kit, we shuffled into the airfield at Windsor. Sitting in the wooden building we only half listened to the corporal giving us our introductory address. Then suddenly his words struck home.

'There's one other thing,' he said. 'Remember to wear your identity discs at all times. We had two prangs last week – couple of fellers burned beyond recognition and neither of 'em was wearing his discs. We didn't know who they were.' He spread his hands appealingly. 'This sort of thing makes a lot of work for us, so remember what I've told you.'

In a moment we were all wide awake and listening intently. Probably thinking as I was – that we had only been playing at being airmen up till now.

I looked through the window at the wind sock blowing over the long flat stretch of green, at the scattered aircraft, the fire tender, the huddle of low wooden huts. The playing was over now. This was where everything started.